GET WELL,
STAY WELL

Barry Gordon, M.D.

GET WELL, STAY WELL

The Successful Patient's Handbook

DEMBNER BOOKS • NEW YORK

Dembner Books
Published by Red Dembner Enterprises Corp., 80 Eighth Avenue, New York, N.Y. 10011
Distributed by W. W. Norton & Company, Inc., 500 Fifth Avenue, New York, N.Y. 10110

Library of Congress Cataloging in Publication Data

Gordon, E. Barry.
    Get well, stay well.

    Includes index.
        1. Medicine, Popular.   2. Patient education.
3. Physician and patient.   I. Title.
RC82.G62   1988   616   87-30601
ISBN 0-942637-02-X

CONTENTS

ACKNOWLEDGMENTS

The following persons have been kind enough to review portions of this work in manuscript: Martin Bernstein, M.D.; Harold Berson, M.D.; Philip Calderone, M.D.; Harvey Dosik, M.D.; Edward Goldstein, M.D.; George Gusset, M.D.; S. Ramachandran Nair, M.D.; Irwin Nelson, M.D.; Stanley Newhouse, M.D.; H. Barry Opell, M.D.; Elliot Senderoff, M.D. Their advice and suggestions have strengthened the book, and I am sincerely indebted to each of them. Needless to say, for controversial statements and any weaknesses that may be found here, they are blameless. The responsibility is mine alone.

I would also like to acknowledge my debt to the late Dr. Robert D. Tick, who encouraged me to pursue my writing from the beginning.

Above all, I am grateful to Elyse Gordon, my wife, for her generous assistance and unwavering support.

ACKNOWLEDGMENTS

CHAPTER 1

INTRODUCTION

Success and failure are terms usually first applied to us while we are students, and then later in life when we go out into the world and find a job, open a business, marry, or enter into other endeavors. They are not commonly used words to describe us when we, inevitably, find ourselves one day becoming a patient. At first thought, you may think that I am refcrring to whether we, as patients, recover or die, but those eventualities have little directly to do with the subject of this book. A successful patient is, very simply, one who gets the greatest possible benefit from the medical profession. Most people do not score an A on being a patient. They derive something less than the most possible from the world of medicine because of their lack of knowledge or misunderstanding of simple concepts. After all, how can you succeed as a patient if you have never been taught how to be one? That is the purpose of this book, to teach you how to be an expert patient, to teach you how to derive the maximum possible benefit, and at the lowest possible cost. I use the word *cost* here in a broad sense, meaning dollar cost to yourself and your insurance carriers, as well as the amount of time you spend either not feeling well or visiting doctors.

One digression before we proceed. I will use the pronoun *he* throughout this book in reference to a physician. This is not because of any chauvinism on my part, but only because of the lack of a suitable English pronoun to refer to both sexes, and to avoid a repetetive *he/she*.

Female physicians are certainly every bit as capable, or noncapable, as their male colleagues.

Some people seem to have an underlying assumption that all they have to do for their health problem is to present themselves to a physician. He will work his magic, find out what is wrong, and fix it. If you assume such an extremely passive posture, you may find success, but it will quite likely be by accident. A lack of understanding of physicians, medical tests, treatments, and fundamental concepts of common illnesses leaves you wide open for failure at each and every phase of being a patient. You may see the wrong physician, one who is marginally competent or even incompetent, or one who is "excessively" interested in making money. You will very likely not be able to tell your doctor accurately what your problem is. You may be subjected to expensive and unnecessary tests. And at the end of it all, you will probably not gain the maximum possible benefit from his advice. You may create major problems out of minor ones, and chronic conditions out of ones that should have been satisfactorily resolved.

Success as a patient requires your very active participation. You have to pick the right physician. That requires a basic knowledge of physicians, as well as some insight in order to judge their ability. You have to tell him your symptoms, something most patients cannot do perfectly, and some cannot do at all! Finally, you have to follow his advice, and if you are to gain the greatest possible benefit from that, you should have a fundamental understanding of diagnostic tests, medications, and those common ailments we fall victim to.

Since picking a physician was listed first, and since you are reading a book about medicine written by one, this seems to be an appropriate place for you to learn a little about the author.

I am an internist and hematologist. I have been in private practice for eighteen years; have been a part-time chief of hematology at a teaching hospital; and have taught house staff in several hospitals, and medical students at a medical school. If this does not paint a clear picture in your mind, you are not unusual. You will understand it better later.

The point I would like to make here is that I have spent portions of my professional life on both sides of three fences. I have been in both private practice and the academic world of medicine. I am functioning both as a primary care physician (local family doctor) and as a specialist to whom other physicians refer patients. I have practiced medicine as part of a group, in a clinic setting, and as a solo practitioner. While all this is not necessarily unique, it does give me a broad view and perspective of the profession. My drawbacks are that I have put a lot of personal opinion in this book (many statements will be, to varying degrees, controversial), and since I am an internist and hematologist practicing in the northeastern United States, I can only see the world of medicine and patients from that perspective.

Throughout this book I present stories and examples to make points. It is very difficult to do that without giving the impression that I am an all-knowing, infallible genius adrift in a world of morons. Such is not my intention, and certainly not the case.

I must also state what this book is *not*. It is not intended to be a medical text for the public. It is not a manual on self-diagnosis and treatment. The purpose is not to make you into an amateur doctor. Only the most common conditions are discussed. The vast majority of diseases are not even mentioned. The many, many exceptions to the general rules are not included.

As in most professions, the amateur, no matter how bright and dedicated, suffers from not knowing what he does not know. It has been my experience that a patient gains little, if any, insight into his or her illness from studying medical texts prepared for the layman. Checking lists of symptoms and physical findings leads more to confusion than understanding. Symptoms may be very similar for a number of different conditions. The body has only a limited number of ways to react to disease. Fever, chills, sweats, loss of appetite, weight loss, and a pain in the abdomen could be due to dozens of different diseases. It is often difficult enough for a physician to make the distinctions. An experienced and talented physician does not make an accurate diagnosis based upon those superficial words that describe symptoms, but rather on their relative degree and on subtle nuances that make up the whole picture. I therefore warn you to not make assumptions that symptoms you may have are due to any disease mentioned in this book. If you do so and you turn out to be wrong, you may make matters worse.

This book is divided into two basic parts. The first, beginning with the next chapter, is meant to give you a working knowledge of physicians, the structure of their profession, and how they make a diagnosis. You should, simultaneously, gain enough insight to determine if your doctor is a "good doctor." You will also be introduced to the world of medical tests, what they mean, the information to be gained from them, and their limitations. You will learn about medications, the purpose of taking them, some fundamental concepts of their types, and some specifics of those most commonly prescribed. You will also learn something about hospitals, and, I hope, rid yourself of some common misconceptions.

The second part deals with diseases and conditions, again, not nearly all, just those most common and which seem to cause the greatest confusion among patients. I am not going to discuss those that are uncommon, or with which I have had limited experience.

So, read on, and learn how to be a successful patient.

PART ONE

PART ONE

CHAPTER 2

WHY GO TO A DOCTOR?

Why should anyone visit a physician? The question sounds simple, and indeed the answers are not difficult, but let us clear the air by spelling them out.

I see the profession of medicine as having two functions of equal importance. The first is to delay illness and death as long as possible. The second is to remedy discomfort. There are, therefore, only four reasons to see a doctor. Nothing is bothering you, but you want to be certain you are as healthy as possible. Something is bothering you, and you want to know what it is. Something is bothering you, and you want it made better. You have a chronic ongoing medical problem that requires periodic checking and evaluation. Let us discuss these four reasons separately.

Is there any reason for you to have a routine checkup when you are feeling well? Most emphatically yes! The simple truth of life is that there are many diseases that can be causing absolutely no symptoms, or symptoms that you really are not aware of, yet be doing significant damage to your body. Hypertension (high blood pressure) is certainly the most well known of these. Except in extreme cases, there simply are no symptoms of hypertension until it has caused severe and irreversible damage to the body. This fact has been well publicized in recent years, but I still have patients who cannot, or will not, comprehend that this disease can progressively damage their body while they are feeling fine.

There are others, many others. You can become anemic to a very significant degree without being aware of anything at all, and the cause of that anemia may be a cancer that is curable early, but incurable later. Early malignancies, cancers, of the breast, the prostate, the colon, cause no symptoms, but are often readily detectable, and curable, in the early stages. This above listing is only a drop in the bucket, and anyone who never gets a checkup because he feels well is a fool. If you do not understand any of the above, reread this after you have finished the book.

That brings up the question of how often you should see a doctor for a routine checkup when you are feeling well. There can be no universally agreed-upon schedule, but certainly it is related to age. The fact is simply that the older you are, the more likely it is that something will go wrong, and sooner rather than later. I have no rigid routine, but the following I believe to be approximate and realistic. Once every three to four years or so is sufficient for someone below forty, every other year up to fifty, yearly up to sixty-five, and twice yearly after that.

The second reason for seeing a doctor, one that very few patients express, is certainly a valid one. Perhaps you have a slight pain or discomfort somewhere. It does not bother you enough to warrant taking medication; you just want to know that it is not something serious, or something that will get worse. If that is the case, tell your physician so. Do not waste your time and his while he writes out a prescription for medication you do not intend to take.

The third reason for seeing a physician is the obvious and most common one. When you feel sick, you want to be made better. There is no time when it is more important to be a successful patient.

The ability of the human mind to bury itself in the sand is indeed wondrous. I am referring to those patients who know that they have a chronic disease or condition, who may be taking multiple medications for it, yet blissfully let years go by without ever having their illness checked by a physician. Concepts such as disease progression, changes due to age, side effects of medications, are completely lost on them. I am reminded of one woman in her fifties (she had not been to a doctor in decades) who was feeling quite ill when she first came to see me. It was no wonder. She had severe hypertension, hypertensive heart disease, was in congestive heart failure, and had uncontrolled diabetes. She was not far removed from death's door. Needless to say, I prescribed quite a few medications. She called me a few days later to learn about her blood tests, told me she was feeling a little better, and that was it! I was reminded of her a year later when her pharmacy called because she wanted her prescriptions renewed! The point is that here was a relatively young woman who was certainly doing everything she could to derive the *least* possible benefit from the profession of medicine. Her hypertension, her heart disease, and her diabetes could each be expected to take years off her life unless brought under "optimal" control, yet she was settling for "feeling a little better." If you have a condition that is chronic, if you are taking medication, see your doctor regularly. The frequency of such follow-up visits depends upon the nature of your problem, but it usually does not have to be more than a few times a year.

I would like to complete this chapter by discussing two commonly used phrases in medicine, phrases I dislike. I have sincere difficulty with the concept of "saving someone's life," and with the term "preventive medicine." They contain implications that are divorced from reality. The facts of life are that everyone is going to die, and if it is not from an accident, murder, or suicide, then it is going to be from a disease. Saving someone's life is really "delaying death." Likewise, most of us are going to die from diseases that are not (at least not yet) preventable. They might, if we are lucky, be "delayable." Some may feel that I am only arguing semantics, but I think that the use of those frequently uttered terms imparts an unrealistic outlook on life in general, and on medicine in particular.

CHAPTER 3

THE PHYSICIAN

Now that you might have made up your mind to see a physician, you have another decision to make. You have to choose the one you want to visit. Seeing the correct or appropriate doctor seems to be a rather haphazard, hit-or-miss proposition for most people, a matter of blind luck, but it need not be.

There are important things you should know about doctors and the world of medicine before making your choice. You should understand what kinds of physicians there are and which kind is appropriate for your problem. Above all, you should have some understanding of the answer to that all-important question: "What is a 'good doctor'?"

Many of my patients do not know that I am an internist, nor even what that word means. Most do not know that I am also a hematologist, and few people really understand exactly what that subspecialty deals with. A patient recently told me that her family wanted her to see an internist, but she decided to come to me first! I asked her what an internist was. She had no idea. On several occasions I have had patients come to see me as a hematologist because of some abnormality with one of their blood tests, an abnormality that had nothing at all to do with the field of hematology.

Perhaps the first thing to understand about types of physicians are two basic terms. These two words divide the world of medicine, physicians, diseases, and even care and treatment, into two fundamental categories. These two words are *medical* and *surgical.*

Medical diseases or conditions are those in which surgery is either not a treatment, or is a treatment of last resort. A few examples where surgery plays no role at all include diabetes, colds, asthma, and most cases of hypertension. Examples where surgery is sometimes used include arteriosclerosis (hardening of the arteries), and gastric (stomach) or duodenal ulcers. In these conditions, medical management and treatment, such as diet and medication, is the treatment of first choice. Surgery only comes into play if medical therapy becomes inadequate or fails.

Surgical diseases are those in which surgery is the only effective treatment. This may be the situation at the onset of the problem, such as with acute appendicitis or many tumors. In other instances, as mentioned above, a medical disease becomes a surgical disease, such as with a duodenal ulcer that perforates (bores a hole through the intestinal wall), or with severe angina (heart pain) that cannot be controlled with medication and requires coronary artery bypass surgery.

Let us digress for a moment to review the basic process leading to the making of a physician. A person becomes a physician upon graduation from medical school, when he earns the M.D. degree. This degree, however, is not enough to obtain a license to practice medicine. A new M.D. has to spend one more year in training, learning and gaining experience in a hospital. This, historically, has been called an internship. Modern times have seen the elimination of the internship in many training programs. New medical school graduates often proceed directly into a residency. That is explained below. In the past, the internship year involved spending three months training in each of the four great branches of medicine, namely medicine and pediatrics, the medical branches, and surgery and obstetrics/gynecology, the surgical ones.

A physician who completes one year of internship is now a general practitioner. Most physicians today, however, become specialists. That requires more years of training, a residency, in their chosen field.

Another way to classify physicians is into those who provide "primary care" and those who practice "specialties." A primary care physician is another term for your regular doctor, the first one you go to when you feel ill, the one who knows you and your body. Many physicians, such as myself, practice both as a primary care physician and as a specialist.

There are basically four kinds of doctors that function as primary care physicians. They are general practitioners, family care specialists, pediatricians, and internists. A general practitioner has already been described. A family care specialist is a doctor who has received additional training in all phases of medicine, sort of like having extra years of internship. A pediatrician has received added years of training in the medical care (as opposed to surgical care) of infants and children. An internist has received additional training in internal medicine, a poor and misleading label. He has undergone additional years of training in the medical care of adults, and functions in a similar manner for them as a pediatrician does for children.

Many physicians who become specialists in internal medicine, and some in pediatrics, continue their training and "subspecialize." The subspecialties, or branches, of internal medicine include:

cardiology: diseases of the heart
gastroenterology: diseases of the esophagus, stomach, intestines, and liver
hematology: diseases of blood cells, bone marrow, and lymph glands, and bleeding disorders
endocrinology: hormonal disorders of glands such as the thyroid, adrenals, pituitary, testes, and ovaries, and diabetes
rheumatology: arthritis and related diseases
nephrology: medical diseases of the kidneys, and dialysis
pulmonary specialists: medical diseases of the lungs such as asthma and emphysema

Remember, all these subspecialists have first become internists. Some function as both primary care physicians and specialists in their particular field, and none are surgeons.

There is similar specialization in the surgical fields. A physician completing a surgical residency will be a general surgeon. Additional years of training will lead to specialization in chest surgery, heart surgery, vascular surgery, neurosurgery, plastic surgery, or orthopedic surgery. Some surgeons will specialize in a very limited field (in breast surgery, for example), but this is usually by choice and not from a specific training program. Other types of surgical training programs include gynecology (surgery on the uterus, vagina, ovaries) and obstetrics, and urology (surgery on the kidneys, urinary bladder, testes, prostate).

Many patients are confused by the existence of medical and surgical specialists in the same field. Examples of this are cardiologists (medical) and cardiac surgeons (surgical); a nephrologist (medical) and a urologist (surgical); a specialist in pulmonary (lung) diseases and a chest surgeon; a neurologist and a neurosurgeon. In the first example, the cardiologist specializes in the medical diagnosis and medical (as opposed to surgical) treatment of heart diseases. If the condition is past the point of medical care, the cardiac surgeon operates. In the second example, although both the nephrologist and urologist are kidney specialists, they deal with entirely different kinds of diseases. The nephrologist specializes in the care of medical diseases of the kidneys, conditions in which surgery plays no role. The urologist cares for surgical diseases, tumors and enlarged prostates for example, which may require operative intervention. I once had a patient who gave me a history of having had some form of nephritis, in her case a serious noninfectious inflammation of the kidneys. Acting on advice from a friend, she went to see a well-known urologist, a surgeon whose specialty has nothing at all to do with her condition. She wasted her time, and her money.

I will again digress for a moment to state my feelings about friends and family. It is almost uncanny how wrong those people can be. In eighteen years of practicing medicine I can count on the fingers of one hand the number of times that "a friend" or "they" or "someone" has ever given a patient of mine correct advice. The surest way to do the wrong thing, and to become more worried, is to discuss the particulars of your problem with friends or family. A woman recently came to me complaining of pain in her leg. She had a degree of superficial phlebitis (clots and inflammation in the veins under the skin). I explained her problem to her and prescribed treatment. The woman spoke to her friends who informed her of all the serious complications of deep-vein phlebitis, a totally different problem. She became so distraught that she almost had a nervous breakdown! If you must discuss your illness with somebody, at least do not listen to anything they have to say. You are rarely, if ever, going to hear anything true.

Let us finish our discussion of the kinds of physicians. Radiologists are specialists in performing and interpreting X-rays, sonograms, scans, and similar diagnostic tests. They function as highly important advisors to physicians directly caring for the patient, and other than in the administration of X-ray or cobalt therapy, play little other direct role in medical care.

Dermatologists are specialists who deal with skin disorders. Dermatology is a separate medical discipline from internal medicine. The surgical aspects are mostly limited to skin biopsies.

Physiatrists are specialists in physical therapy and rehabilitation.

Neurologists are specialists in diseases of the brain, spinal cord, and nerves.

Psychiatrists are specialists who deal with disorders of the mind. Many people are confused as to the difference between a psychiatrist and a psychologist. A psychiatrist is an M.D. A psychologist is not. Both deal with the more routine kinds of mental problems such as unwarranted anxiety, and personality and behavior disorders. The psychiatrist, however, is the one who cares for those who are frankly psychotic (really crazy).

Pathology is the general study of the nature, origin, and course of disease. The pathologist usually doesn't "see" patients, at least not while they are alive. He is the one who performs autopsies and examines biopsied tissues or fluids. He has the final word on what disease is present when a biopsy is necessary to make a diagnosis.

Now that you have some understanding of the kinds of physicians, who do you go to when you do not feel well? I firmly believe that everyone should have a primary care physician. There is sometimes a danger in going directly to a practicing specialist, a physician who ordinarily sees patients with only certain kinds of diseases. That danger is caused by "tunnel vision," the natural inclination and habit many specialists have of looking for illnesses primarily in their field of specialty. Do not think that this phenomenon is unusual or unimportant. If your particular problem is not in his field of specialty, there may be an unnecessary delay in making the diagnosis, or a completely erroneous diagnosis. I once saw a patient in hematologic consultation whose main complaint was pain in the upper left part of his abdomen. The man had first consulted a very competent gastroenterologist. He had undergone an upper G.I. series, and was scheduled for other tests, when he decided to visit his general practitioner. That physician found that the patient's spleen was enlarged and was the source of his pain, and referred him to me. It can certainly be argued, and rightfully so, that the first physician should have detected the enlarged and tender spleen, but the facts of everyday medical life are that doctors are only human, and specialists have a strong tendency to look first for diseases in their own specialty.

I recently examined a woman who was visiting from another state and had never been my patient. Several points are illustrated by this elderly woman who sees a gastroenterologist and a cardiologist, both of whom limit their practice to their specialty. Her first comment to me after my examination was: "Nobody ever examines me like that!" Her remark did not surprise me at all, even though I had only done a simple routine examination. She is seeing two physicians who are primarily interested in their own fields. Her inability to obtain a complete physical examination is not entirely their fault, it is partially hers. But that is not the end of her story. She sees the gastroenterologist because she has a hiatus hernia and has occasional heartburn, and the cardiologist because she has slight angina. Both of these are very elementary and uncomplicated medical conditions. She needs the ongoing care of those specialists as much as you need a plumber to turn on your kitchen sink faucet, or an electrician to turn on your lights. What she needs is a primary care physician who cares for *all* of her. Many patients, in their ignorance, decide they need specialists, so-called top men, to care for routine and uncomplicated medical problems, then suffer medical neglect. It is not at all uncommon. But there is still one more point to be made concerning this woman. Her primary complaint to me was that she keeps "spitting up." She had complained about this to her gastroenterologist, who promptly sent her for a whole series of X-rays, and later told her that she had esophageal dysfunction, meaning that something was wrong with her swallowing mechanism. I asked her what she meant by "spitting up," if she was actually regurgitating food she swallowed. She emphatically stated that that was not the case. As a matter of fact, she seemed surprised to learn what esophageal dysfunction, the term she had just used, actually meant! After several more minutes, and a demonstration by her, it finally became evident that what she really meant was that she was clearing her throat, and that her problem was a simple postnasal drip! Perhaps now you understand what I mean by "tunnel vision."

That brings to mind a patient from many years ago who complained of recurrent mild chest pain. She also had seen a gastroenterologist on her own. The physician found esophageal spasm during fluoroscopic X-rays and blamed that for her occasional symptoms. Treatment for this condition, however, had not brought relief. I asked her if she had experienced her chest discomfort at the time the doctor had seen the spasm. She answered no, then looked at me with the funniest expression, stating that she had never thought about that before! It turned out that she had mild angina, and treatment for that condition eliminated her symptoms. I have not seen her since. She is probably going to a cardiologist!

To be sure, I do not mean to pick on gastroenterologists exclusively. These and the following are simply some of the many incidents that come to mind.

A long-time patient of mine was vacationing in another state. He experienced increasingly severe pain in a leg and on the advice of a friend went directly to see an orthopedist. The orthopedist examined his leg, took X-rays, and prescribed arthritis pills. The pain grew worse and the patient flew home to see me. One feel of his ice-cold foot revealed that he had developed a totally blocked artery. Subsequent surgery saved the leg. The finding of an almost totally bloodless foot does not require any extraordinary degree of medical skill, and, certainly, the orthopedist should have detected it. The practical point, however, is that my patient went to a physician who, by human force of habit, immediately thinks of bones and joints. The fact that doctors are only human will be repeated again and again throughout this book.

Specialists are an integral and exceedingly important part of medicine. I am one for blood diseases, and I use the services of others frequently, but patients should be aware of the danger of tunnel vision. Have a primary care physician who knows you, one whom you trust. See him first. He will likely be less expensive. He will not have the tunnel vision habit since he is used to seeing all manner of illnesses. He can diagnose and care for the great bulk of medical problems, and is the one to decide if a medical or surgical specialist is necessary. If you do need one, he can direct you to a specialist he knows is competent and will not perform unnecessary tests. I will have more to say about physician referral to specialists below.

Let us now examine the concept of the "good doctor."

We all, usually unfortunately, have to seek advice from professionals on occasions during our lives. If we think about it for a moment, we must realize that all professions have their share of those who are extremely capable, those adequate, those marginally competent, and those frankly incompetent. It is difficult, to say the least, for the lay person, no matter how intelligent or well educated, to be able to judge the ability of the professional he engages. When it comes to physicians, a poor choice can mean needless suffering or far worse. I cannot lay out a rigid set of guidelines for patients to refer to when trying to evaluate the competency of their doctor. There are some considerations below. I do believe, however, that a considered and thoughtful reading of this book will enable you to make a fairly accurate judgment of the physician you visit.

What *is* a good doctor? There is a simple answer to that question. It is a physician who finds out what is causing your complaints and prescribes the proper treatment, and one who finds things that are wrong with you even if they are not causing any symptoms.

What qualities *make* a physician a good doctor is not as simple to answer.

Knowledge—a good grasp of the fundamentals of medicine and the basic sciences—is essential to being a good physician. No one, however, knows everything. That is an impossibility. Therefore, it is also very important for a physician to know what he does not know, to be able to judge when the services of a specialist are needed. To what extremes can this question of knowledge be taken? I have known physicians who were encyclopedias of medical knowledge, but could not begin to apply it to the everyday task of taking care of patients. A given symptom may theoretically be caused by dozens, or even hundreds, of diseases, most usually quite rare. The remembrance of the list alone is insufficient to make a good doctor. On the other hand, I once knew a physician who was appallingly ignorant of medicine. He did, however, constantly send his patients to specialists, and as a result they all received good medical care. Was he a good doctor? Knowledge, whether it is meager or great, by itself is of little value if it is not applied, and there are two important qualities in a physician necessary for that application.

The first, and least important of the two, is simply talent, a nose for disease or illness, an intuitive feel for what is going on in a patient's body, the extra sense that makes one bellyache different from the other ten. It cannot be taught. It is either there or not.

The second quality is far more important. It has been called dedication, but a better term, I think, is interest—the time, the extra minutes, given to thought, to an attention to detail, to have a determination to be reasonably thorough and not overlook anything. *Time* is the key word. I believe the single most important attribute to the making of a "good doctor" is the time he spends in both consideration and conversation. The time spent evaluating a patient is the most important and most valuable element in making a diagnosis. Treatment, feeling better, being as healthy as possible, living as long as possible, all have to begin with a correct diagnosis. The importance of this aspect of time will become more apparent in Chapter 4.

Time is also one of the essential ingredients in the establishment of a relationship between the physician and his patient, for the generation of a feeling of confidence. As much as we need the best possible medical care from our doctor, we also need to have a strong feeling of confidence in him. That is not only essential for our psychological and emotional comfort and well being, but it also plays a great role in the healing process of physical diseases. We humans all become frightened children when faced with the prospect of illness and death. I am seeing a woman in the hospital now. She is one hundred and two years old, yet she keeps crying out for her mother. I believe it is a very important function of a physician to take the time to be emotionally supportive, to be his patient's friend, his parent, to help alleviate the fears and anxieties that accompany illness.

What you want, therefore, is a physician with knowledge, a detective's nose for illness, and, above all else, an interest in his patients. How do you find them? How do you know you can trust the one you choose? How do you know he is competent?

It is easiest to find specialists. Certainly, the best way is to be referred to one by another physician with ability. Generally speaking, physicians of equal ability refer to each other. The referring physician either wants his patient cared for properly or is seeking advice, and neither would be obtained by the services of anyone he considers to be an inferior. Yet, it has been a very common phenomenon during my professional life for me to recommend a specific specialist to a patient only to find out that he went to another who was recommended by "someone." To this day I cannot comprehend why a person would entrust his health to me for years, yet ignore my professional recommendations as to the ability of another physician. Most of the time, these other physicians were capable, but on occasion my patients would wind up seeing a total incompetent, sometimes with unfortunate results.

Referral by another physician is the best method to find a specialist, but how do you find your primary care physician? Certainly *not* by the recommendations of "a friend," "someone," or "they" *alone*. These nonprofessional recommendations may be a place to start, but you will be far better off if you assume that your friend or relative is not an expert judge of doctors and decide for yourself, from what you learn in this book. You are not going to find a "perfect" doctor. Doctors are all human, therefore by definition imperfect, less than ideal. I believe that the kind I describe as being good doctors can be found, but that, unfortunately, they are becoming fewer in number as the profession of medicine continues its ongoing change under governmental and economic pressures that encourage physicians to become, more and more, collators of laboratory tests, and to spend less and less time with their patients.

I believe that there is nothing more important than having a single, interested, capable, personal, primary care physician to take care of you. If this responsibility is split up among more than one physician, as it often is in group and clinic settings, something is inevitably lost. That something is both the human interaction between patient and physician, and some of the medical knowledge about you and your body. The recording of findings and impressions in a chart, no matter how complete and legibly written, is not the same as seeing the same physician each time you need a doctor.

There is one more factor to consider when choosing a doctor, either primary care physician or specialist, and that is his location. Many people choose to travel some distance, to the "city," to a major center to see a "big man." The simple fact is that *there are only two kinds of doctors, the ones who know what they are doing, and the ones who do not.* Except for some rare or complicated disease, or unusual kinds of surgery, going to the "city" does not guarantee that you will get the best care. There are no significant forces at work in our society that push good doctors to the urban centers and marginal ones to the suburbs or country. There are disadvantages, however, to using doctors who are far away. If you require hospitalization, it will be difficult for friends and family to visit you. If an emergency arises you might need immediate care, and there will be no local physician who knows you. If you have a chronic condition that worsens, or if you become partially incapacitated for any reason, you might find it difficult to travel a great distance to your doctor. There is one more point to consider. A local physician may not want to be bothered with taking care of someone else's patient, nor may he want to start to take care of a patient near the end of a long illness. If he does, it may likely be with reluctance and annoyance.

CHAPTER 4

BEFORE THE OFFICE VISIT

Y ou have decided to see a physician either because you have symptoms or want a checkup. You have received the name of a doctor from family or friends. You have called and made an appointment. You have, it is hoped, even found out what kind of physician he is. Is that all you need do? *No!* Now you have to prepare to succeed at what many, many patients fail at, *telling your doctor what is wrong with you.*

The first several minutes of contact between you and your physician are going to be spent on your medical history, the details of the current symptoms, and the recitation of your past medical problems. Despite the proliferation of blood tests, scans, and other diagnostic tools, *the history of the patient, of the symptoms and illness, as presented by the patient and elicited by the physician, is still, by far, the most important factor in the making of a diagnosis.* The all-importance of the history of the patient is what physicians are taught in medical school, and what we learn for ourselves through experience. I think you would be hard put to find a physician who disagrees with that philosophy. This is not to say that modern diagnostic testing is unimportant or without value, because that is certainly not the case, but rather that those tests are far more limited in their specificity, accuracy, and sensitivity than most patients suspect. Those aspects of diagnostic testing will be discussed later in the book.

This history taking then, this most important source of information your doctor will have about your illness, is going to come directly from you. It only makes common sense that you should not only have that information, but also be able to present it in an understandable way. It will give you, at the same time, your first, and perhaps most important, clues as to his ability, and his interest. If all your doctor's history-taking consists of is you filling out a form, and nothing more than that, find another doctor.

This crucial first step can become, at one extreme, an irritating experience for both of you. You may wind up feeling tongue-tied and dumb, and your doctor may feel as if he is practicing veterinary medicine (their patients never tell them their symptoms). On the other extreme, you could sit down, tell your story, and have the experience of having your doctor know immediately what is wrong with you. The only thing necessary to prevent the former situation and to promote the latter is for you to simply pay attention to the specifics of exactly what is bothering you.

If you stop to think about it for a minute, and if you accept the fact that doctors are human, then you will realize that you have the ability to either interest the doctor in your case, or bore him with it. Do not begin with broad generalizations or gross exaggerations such as "I don't feel good" or "Everything hurts," and then silence. You will probably make him disinterested, and he may assume there is nothing seriously wrong with you. You should be able to present a fairly precise story and be able to answer his questions. You will not be benefitted if you sit there in confusion, unsure of what you feel or have felt. The time to begin the process of analyzing your complaints is *not* while he is sitting there waiting. It may sound simple, but few patients can do it very well, and some hardly at all. So before you go, while you still have time, learn about symptoms. You may find the following a bit overwhelming. Do not try to memorize it. Just read it over, then keep this book handy for reference before your next visit to the doctor.

Pain is probably the most common symptom, but it is not enough to just say "It hurts here." For all pain, know *exactly* where it hurts. It has not been at all uncommon for patients to tell me that they had a pain in their abdomen but are not certain exactly where it was, or that they had a pain in their back and then proceed to first point to the lumbar area and then the kidneys, uncertain as to where it was.

Know when the pain began, as precisely as you can determine. Know if the pain is the same as when it began or if it is getting worse. Pay attention to whether the pain travels or radiates, and if it is constant or intermittent. If it is intermittent, how long do you feel it? How long does it stay away?

Be specific with the part of the body you identify. A woman once complained to me about her "arthritis" pain, and that she had not experienced relief from the arthritis pills prescribed by another doctor. I asked her where her pain was. She stated the knee, pointing then to a spot on her leg several inches below the knee. The woman had superficial phlebitis, no arthritic pain at all. Certainly the physician she saw first should have made the proper diagnosis, but what would have happened, how much pain, time, and money would she have saved if she had told him that her *leg* hurt? Call a knee a knee, a foot a foot, do not add unnecessary confusion to an already difficult situation.

Do not confuse the words *stomach* and *abdomen*. The stomach is a pouch in the upper abdomen, in the soft area between your ribs. It is part of the gastrointestinal tract and receives swallowed food. The abdomen is the area in front of your body from the lower border of your ribs to the pelvis.

If you have or had pain in the abdomen, where in the abdomen exactly? Is it above or below your belly button, is it central, or left or right? Does it go or radiate anywhere, up or down, left or right, into the chest or back or the groin? If it does go to the back, does it go "around" your body to the back, or "through" your body to the back? Where exactly in the back do you feel it? A variance of just a few inches can be indicative of different conditions. When did it really begin? Often a patient will state that a pain began a week or so ago, and later I find out that it really began a year ago, lasts a week or two, and then goes away for a while.

Is it a constant pain, or does it vary in intensity? Does it come and go, sometimes completely gone? If it is not constant, how long does it last or stay at its worst? How long does it go away or feel better? Does the time of day matter? Is it related in any way to your menstrual cycle?

Does the position of your body matter? Is the area that hurts tender? (Tenderness means that it hurts more when you touch it.) Does eating have any effect on your pain? Does it make it better or worse? If eating does have an effect, when does it happen? As soon as you start eating, a few minutes later, an hour later? Again, if eating does affect the pain, does it matter what you eat? Does moving your bowels or urinating affect the pain, or does the pain make you want to do either of those? Does sexual intercourse affect the pain? When the pain is at its worst, do you want to lie still, or do you move around a lot, squirm? Are there any associated symptoms with the pain such as fever, sweating, nausea, vomiting, belching, heartburn, shortness of breath, flatulence (passing gas)? To a physician these specifics are not just very important; they are *crucial!*

A doctor will want to know similar things about chest pain. Where is it exactly? Does it radiate or go anywhere such as your neck, jaw, teeth, back, abdomen, shoulder, or arm? What kind of pain is it? Is it sticking, stabbing, burning, pressing, squeezing? Does regular breathing make it worse? Does deep breathing or coughing make it worse? Have you been coughing? Does the movement of your body affect the pain? If you move or swing your arms, is it worse? Is the area tender, does it hurt more if you touch it? If you are not sure, press on it!

If you have pain in an arm or a leg, where exactly is it? Is it in a joint? Is the area tender to the touch? Has it ever been red or swollen as compared to the one on the other side? Does lying, sitting, standing, walking affect it? If it happens when you walk, how far? Will the pain go away if you stand still? If you sit? If you lie down?

If the pain is in a joint or joints, which joints? If it is in a hand or finger, which joints and which fingers? Know which fingers specifically bother you; certain conditions will affect some fingers and not others. Look at your fingers, and notice that each has *two* joints. Different kinds of arthritis affect different joints, so know which specific joints hurt.

If it is your back that is bothering you, where exactly does it hurt, and since when? If you point to a spot just two or three inches from where you actually felt or feel it, you are going to mislead your doctor. Does breathing, coughing, eating, urinating, moving your bowels affect it? Does the pain go anywhere, around to the front, to your groin, into a buttock, down a leg? Which part of the leg? Does the position of your body make a difference? What time of day is it worst? How does it feel in the morning? Did you lift or move something heavy?

Constitutional symptoms refer to the general condition of your health. Has your appetite been affected? Your thirst? If your doctor asks you "How's your appetite?" do not start telling him what you eat! Appetite is the "desire" to eat. And it does not help to say that you have never been a big eater. He wants to know if there has been a *change*. Have you lost any weight? Vague answers do not help. Weigh yourself before you go if you are not sure. Notice if your clothes are looser. Try to know how much weight you have lost, and when the weight loss began. If you have lost your appetite, has there been any nausea? What happens if you do eat? What do you feel?

Have you had any fever, chills, or sweating? Take your temperature if you feel warm. Take it an hour or so after a chill. Are you sweating more than normal? More than can be accounted for by the temperature and your activity? The usual sequence is chills, then fever, then sweating. Are you more tired than normal, more than you were a year ago? Do you become fatigued more easily?

If you are coughing, are you bringing up any phlegm? If so, what color? Look at it! If you have phlegm, are you coughing it up or just clearing your throat? Pay attention. I think I have had more problem with the words *spitting up* than anything else. It is amazing that some patients will use the same expression for vomiting, coughing up something from the lungs, and clearing the throat. Do not be careless when you describe these symptoms.

If you have urinary symptoms such as pain, burning, or discomfort when urinating, mention it even if it is minimal, and pay attention to the following: When did it begin? Did it ever happen before? If a male, is there any discharge from the penis; if a female, from the vagina? Both of you, look at your underwear. Any stains? How often do you have to urinate during the day, during the night? Count the number of times and write it down! Do you have to go in a hurry or can you hold it in? Pay attention to the force of the urinary stream. Is it a strong steady flow or does it dribble or trickle? How much urine comes out each time? Are you just urinating smaller amounts more frequently, or passing a greater quantity of urine? Pay attention! Look at the color of the urine. Any change? Any discomfort associated with sex?

Has there been any change in your bowel habits? Do you go less often, more often, how often? Has there been any change in the color, the consistency? Look! Is there pain or discomfort associated with it? Where? Do you see any mucus, blood? Look! There are many, many people who simply do not ever look in a toilet bowl. Do not be one of them.

Shortness of breath (dyspnea) is a very common complaint and has many different causes. Before you see a doctor, take five minutes to learn more about your particular shortness of breath. Are you really feeling a shortness of breath or are you experiencing a feeling of weakness, or a feeling of heaviness or tightness in the chest? Is your breathing heavy? Are you panting? When does this shortness of breath occur? Does it happen only with exertion such as walking, and if so, how far? Ten steps? Ten blocks? Or does it happen even if you are resting, sitting? How long does it last? Is there any pain, palpitations, dizziness, or other discomfort associated with it? How long ago did your shortness of breath begin? A week? A month? Five years? Is it getting worse, or is it more or less the same as when it started?

Dizziness is another common complaint of many patients, but again, you have to pay attention to the specifics. What exactly do you mean by dizzy? Do you feel as if you are going to faint, black out? Is it a sense of loss of balance that you feel? Maybe you mean a feeling of light-headedness? Is it constant or intermittent, and if the latter, when exactly does it occur? Does it happen only when you stand up from a lying or sitting position, or when you move your head no matter the position of your body? Patients will often tell me they get dizzy when they bend over, but further questioning reveals that they are unsure if it happens when they bend over, or really when they straighten up!

This has been by no means an exhaustive list of symptoms. Try to pay attention to everything before you go to the doctor. It will make his work, the finding out of what is wrong with you, much easier and quicker. It should also serve you as a guide as to what should be asked by a physician, depending upon what your complaints are.

There are other kinds of questions that should be asked by a physician, again depending upon the nature of the patient's complaints. I am referring to inquiring into a patient's current family or work circumstances. It is not at all uncommon for a simple general question of that nature to provoke a quivering face and tears, followed by an outpouring of problems the individual has been trying to cope with. The underlying emotional basis for the patient's physical symptoms not only becomes quite evident, but a few minutes of allowing a patient to vent what he or she has been holding inside may be the most important and effective therapy the physician can provide.

It should now be quite evident that the making of a diagnosis requires *time*. If something is wrong with your car, a mechanic can hook it up to his diagnostic machinery and find the problem. But humans are not cars. Not only are their workings far more complex, but there is an emotional overlay to everything. We could, I suppose, develop a system of medicine where every patient, for every symptom he lists, automatically has every conceivable test done. That would eliminate the need for a physician to spend his time asking questions and giving considered thought to his patient's problem. He could function in the manner of a technician, using a computer to collate all the laboratory findings. I think such a system would work, but not well, and it certainly would be very, very costly. Yet, again unfortunately, that is the direction medicine today is headed. Physicians are being paid far more for whatever tests and procedures they can devise than for the time they give to their patients. Yet, the reward to the patient from the latter is far more substantial than that from the former. There is more on this aspect of the emphasis and costs of medicine in Chapter 7.

There are other things you should do before your visit to the doctor's office. First, write down everything of significance that is bothering you. If you come up with an excessively long list, however, you may overload your doctor. My advice is that if there is nothing really new bothering you (all your complaints are rather chronic), and you are basically going for a checkup, tell him everything. If, however, you have a new symptom or complaint that prompted you to make the visit in the first place, concentrate on that. Leave your ten-year-old backache for another time. Also write down your past history, any major illnesses, hospitalizations, and surgery. Either write a list of all your medications and dosage strengths (which are on the labels), or bring along all your bottles. A patient of mine taking an anticoagulant developed a severe pain in his elbow and went directly to an orthopedist, neglecting to tell him about the medication he was taking. The orthopedist diagnosed arthritis and prescribed medication. After several more days of severe pain, the patient came to see me. He was hemorrhaging into the joint. The orthopedist should have made the diagnosis, but the patient also made mistakes. He went to a specialist on his own, and then did not tell him about very potent medication he was taking. Remember, physicians in practice for decades begin to forget what it is like to not be a doctor. There is a human tendency to begin to take things for granted, such as patients telling him when they are taking an important medication like an anticoagulant. If you expect robotlike perfection from the profession of medicine, you are going to be disappointed.

As a general rule, do not eat before going to the doctor, although drinking water is all right. He may want to do blood tests, especially if it is your first visit or you have not seen him in a while. The normal values of some blood tests are based upon a fasting condition. That is especially true for sugar, cholesterol, and triglycerides. If you are going to see your doctor in the morning, do not eat at all that day. If your visit is scheduled for the afternoon or evening, call and ask him or his office assistant what you should do.

Be able to provide a urine specimen. How many times patients have told me they just urinated, and then have to drink water and wait, or have to come back a second time.

It is fine to take a shower or a bath, please do, but do not douche, especially not if you have a vaginal problem. You may be washing away what your doctor needs to make a diagnosis.

Do not cover a rash with medication so it cannot be seen.

I also want my patients to take all their regular medications before they come to the office. If continuing medication is necessary, I want to see them with the full effects of what I have prescribed. I frequently have the frustrating experience of having a patient that I have begun treating for a chronic condition, such as high blood pressure or diabetes, come to the office with the following story: "I ran out of my pills last week and wanted to see you before I refilled them." This is a classic example of a waste of time. I already know what the patient's blood pressure or sugar is without medication, and these conditions just do not go away except under unusual circumstances. I now want to know what the medication is doing for them, but they have not taken it for a week and the effect is gone! If you really want to know if you can do without your medication, speak to your doctor about it first, but otherwise do not discontinue taking your medication before you see him.

CHAPTER 5

DURING THE OFFICE VISIT

If you have made an appointment to see a doctor, either keep it or call beforehand to cancel. If you keep it, show up on time, not early or late. There are some physicians who do not care how long their patients have to wait, but most who work by appointment try to prevent long periods of sitting in their waiting rooms. Emergencies do arise, however, and often what was expected to be a twenty minute visit becomes an hour. Remember, there may be seriously ill people behind those doors, so try to be a patient patient.

Your first contact with the doctor will be when he takes your history. Do not worry about being nervous or frightened. Most people are, so just accept it and yourself. If you have prepared a list of symptoms, past medical history, and medications you are taking, have it with you. Some physicians have new patients fill out a form for their medical history. There is nothing wrong with that, but if you are seeing someone who is to be your primary care physician, and there is no more to the doctor's history taking than that form, forget him and go somewhere else. *To a doctor who is interested, the manner in which a patient states a complaint is as important as the complaint itself.*

After you have given your history to the doctor and he has finished asking his questions, there is little for you to do except to be aware of what he is doing during his physical examination. It is difficult to outline exactly what he should be doing. The depth of a physical examination is dependent upon your age, when he last examined you, and, of course, your complaints. If you are a new patient, or one who has not been seen for a while, you should be examined from head to toe. If you last saw your doctor a month ago for a complete physical, and now you are there to have your blood pressure rechecked or for a cold, another complete physical may not be necessary. Let us assume that you are fifty years old, are seeing him for the first time, and have nonspecific symptoms. You are feeling kind of tired and run-down lately.

One word of caution. Understand that if I stated that the following is a "complete" physical examination, I would be inundated by outraged physicians crying out that it is totally inadequate. A physician's physical examination can range from one much more complicated and involved than I describe, to one lasting five seconds. What I describe is my concept of an "acceptable" physical examination, and even that will undoubtedly bring the wrath of many down upon my head.

Every patient needs to have his urine tested and weight recorded. This should be done almost every visit. Testing the urine is an easy, inexpensive, and quick way of finding many unexpected conditions. If you are having urinary symptoms, you will also need to have your urine checked microscopically in the office or a laboratory, and you might need a culture. (See Chapter 7: Tests.)

The physical examination usually begins with the patient in the sitting position, and often the blood pressure determination is the first step. If it is normal on the first reading, fine. If it is not normal, and it is not checked again after you have relaxed for a while, do not accept the doctor's diagnosis of hypertension. As a matter of fact, do not accept him! (See Chapter 17: Hypertension.)

Every physician has his own routine for performing a physical examination, and where he begins and ends does not matter. We will start at the top and work our way down.

The eyes should be checked at least to see that there is no jaundice (that the white area is white) and that the red area inside the lower eyelid is not excessively pale. Many physicians will routinely look into the eyes with an ophthalmoscope to check the retina. Others leave that to an ophthalmologist, who is more expert at that type of examination.

The ears may be checked, but it is unlikely anything abnormal will be found if there are no symptoms related to those organs.

The mouth and its contents certainly should be examined (at least a peek) for evidence of precancerous changes and the condition of the teeth. The tongue will show changes in certain vitamin deficiencies. Inability to chew properly can cause a lot of symptoms.

The entire neck area—front, back, and sides—should be felt for the presence of enlarged lymph glands and the presence of an enlarged thyroid or thyroid nodules. Some physicians may feel for the carotid artery pulses, the major arteries to the brain, or may check that the trachea, the windpipe, is in the midline of the body.

All examinations should include feeling for enlarged lymph glands in the armpits, and a check of the arms and hands themselves. A quick check that the pulses in both wrists are fairly equal is indicated if the patient is of an age to have developed hardening of the arteries.

The lungs should at least be listened to, and this includes that part of the lungs that is in the front of the chest on the right side. The corresponding area on the left side is occupied by the heart. This right middle lobe of the lung is a very common area for infection. When your doctor tells you to take a deep breath, do so deeply and through an open mouth. Lungs can also be examined by percussion (thumping with a finger), and by checking for fremitus (vibrations caused by talking). This may not be done if there are no lung problems, but can provide additional information if a lung condition is present.

The heart can be examined and listened to in the upright position, lying down, or both. There are slight differences in what can be heard in different positions.

At this point the patient must lie down for the rest of the examination.

I believe that a woman's breasts should be routinely checked for lumps, and not by gynecologists only. The earlier a tumor can be detected, the better the chance for a cure.

The entire abdomen must be palpated (felt). This includes a check for hernias in the lower abdomen, and for masses or areas of tenderness everywhere. Some areas of the abdomen are normally slightly tender so do not become alarmed unnecessarily. Both the spleen and the liver must be checked for enlargement and tenderness, and proper examination of both require that the patient take in a deep breath. The taking of the breath pushes down the diaphragm, which in turn pushes down the liver, located under the lower right ribs, and the spleen, located under the lower left ribs. When your doctor tells you to take a deep breath, do it through your open mouth. If he does not ask you to take a deep breath when checking the right and left side of the upper abdomen, he is not doing it right. There certainly can be more to the examination of the abdomen than outlined above. Areas can be percussed, parts can be palpated with the body turned in different positions, and the sounds made by the intestines, or by a deformed or blocked major abdominal artery, can be listened to with a stethoscope, especially if there is an abdominal problem.

The groin should be checked for the pulses of the large arteries that enter the legs there, and for hernias and any enlarged lymph glands. We will discuss examination of the sex organs later.

The ankles and lower legs should be checked for edema (accumulation of fluid in the tissues). This is also a good time to see if there is any tenderness in the large leg veins, checked by squeezing the calf muscles upwards. A physican should also note if there are any incipient problems with the lower legs such as superficial phlebitis or skin problems from chronic edema.

The feet should be checked to see if the pulses of the two major arteries there can be felt. A pulse is simply the sudden expansion of an artery, the result of the heart's contraction causing a surge of blood flow. The absence of these pulses may indicate a significant degree of hardening of the arteries in the leg or higher. This can occur without symptoms and does not require treatment, but should you ever develop symptoms, it would be useful to know if the pulses were palpable before.

Rectal examinations are very important, the more so the older you become. It is not uncommon for many of my patients to mutter about this part of the examination. I ignore them. It is one of the best and easiest tests to find common cancers before they have spread. In both sexes the examination will detect tumors within reach of the finger, but more important, it allows the retrieval of a small amount of stool for testing for blood. This chemical testing for blood is very sensitive and can be positive in many conditions that may not be causing symptoms at the moment. This includes tumors from the stomach to the colon that may be bleeding, ulcers, inflammatory disorders, and others. There is another reason for this examination in men. The physician can feel the prostate gland through the rectum and detect infections, enlargement, and tumors.

Examination of the male external sexual organs is most important in the young. Some tumors are more common at that age, and some young men may have an undiagnosed undescended testis. Many women prefer to have a vaginal examination performed by a gynecologist. Others do not want to see another physician for a routine examination and Pap smear when they have no complaints. Likewise, some primary care physicians will do gynecologic examinations, others will not. I personally will do a routine pelvic examination and Pap smear if the patient desires, but will refer her to a gynecologist if there is any problem. I think the best course is for all women to see a gynecologist regularly.

Part of the routine physical may include a portion of a neurological examination such as testing your reflexes and determining if skin sensations are normal.

Other things may be done during your office visit such as an electrocardiogram, chest X-ray, and blood tests. These will be discussed in the chapter on tests.

After the physical examination and any tests performed in the office are completed, you should have a chance to speak with your doctor. I do not believe that a physician's role and responsibility is satisfied by only caring for the physical problem. The emotional state and satisfaction of the patient is also important. In my opinion, if your doctor is not interested enough in you as person to speak with you in private, find another doctor. He should be willing to explain your case to you, and to answer all your questions. You should not expect, however, that he will be willing to answer all your questions more than once. It is annoying to explain something for several minutes only to have the same question asked again a few minutes later. If you are the type that becomes nervous easily and may not be able to remember what he will say to you, bring someone along to listen and help you remember, or have a pen and paper to take notes. If it happens that you do forget something he said that you feel is important, call him up and ask him. Again, if you have the repeated experience of being unable to speak with him on the telephone, get another doctor. This does not mean, however, that you can make a pest of yourself, or call him on a Saturday night for something that could wait for Monday morning. If you are going to call him, have a pencil and paper on hand, and all your medications next to you, so you can jot down what he says and will be able to discuss your medications by name and dosage if that is necessary. Remember, I believe the single most important quality to look for in a physician who is going to be your doctor is *interest*. A physician who is a genius will miss things if he is not interested, while one who is far less knowledgeable will catch them because he will ask seemingly trivial, yet important, questions, and will get help from a specialist if he needs it.

CHAPTER 6

AFTER THE OFFICE VISIT

Now you have either been told that you are in good health, or that something is wrong with you. If it is the latter, then you have been given a diagnosis. Do you understand it? Many physicians feel that the less a patient knows about his illness, the better. I strongly disagree. I believe that it is unlikely you will have success as a patient if you do not fully understand your problem. It is your doctor's obligation and responsibility to see that you do.

Some diagnoses are complete, the name of a disease such as angina due to arteriosclerotic heart disease, or a cancer of the colon. Others have to be amplified to determine the severity or state, such as with diabetes, which can be labeled uncontrolled, diet controlled, insulin dependent, etc. It is not completely necessary to know the medical terms as long as you understand the different degrees of severity, and you know where your problem fits in.

Some diagnoses are terms that signify a "condition," not a disease. A condition is not a complete diagnosis unto itself, but rather is the result of some known or unknown underlying disease process. Congestive heart failure, anemia, gastrointestinal bleeding, and edema are examples of conditions that always have an underlying cause. The importance of finding the underlying cause depends upon what the condition is and its severity. Many times the underlying cause will be found as part of the routine examination and tests. Sometimes additional tests are necessary. Occasionally, the tests necessary to find out for certain are worse than the condition itself.

I think that you should also understand that there are two basic kinds of diagnoses. A "clinical" diagnosis is made on the basis of the history and the physical examination. A "laboratory" diagnosis is made on the basis of tests.

Patients should be aware that there are fads in medical diagnoses just like everything else. Sometimes a diagnosis becomes fashionable, often because some television news reporter needs a story and picks something up from a medical journal. This usually involves the publicizing of a disease or condition that is well known to the medical community, but relatively unknown otherwise. People hear about this condition, think it is something new, or that recent advances have been made, and decide they suffer from it. Physicians are human also, and many have the inclination to blame vague symptoms without obvious cause on whatever diagnosis is "in." Hypoglycemia (low blood sugar) was a fashionable diagnosis during the nineteen seventies, but is not as popular anymore. I know this because I used to have many patients coming into my office for a first visit with a history of a previous diagnosis of hypoglycemia, but I have not seen any new ones in a while. Of course, very few patients such as these really have or had true hypoglycemia. This is not to say that there is no such condition as hypoglycemia—there is, and there are different types and causes—but there are nowhere near the number of cases that used to be diagnosed. One more modern fad is osteoporosis, recent publicized studies supposedly indicating that calcium should be taken to prevent this condition. More will be said about this subject in a later chapter. Remember two things. The most accurate thing to be said about medical studies is that most are doomed to be refuted. Much of what you read in newspapers or magazines, or hear on television, about anything related to health is inaccurate. The stated facts may be correct, but the impression you get from them will more than likely be erroneous.

It may be that your doctor has found a condition that requires follow up, repeated visits to determine if it is under control. It has been my experience that many physicians tell their parents to come back too frequently. Few chronic conditions in medicine change abruptly or drastically in a short period of time. High blood pressure, for example, once it is under control with medication, does not have to be checked more often than every few to several months.

If there has been a diagnosis of some kind, then your doctor has likely prescribed treatment. Now you have your best chance to fail as a patient. One way to increase the probability of failing is to not understand what is wrong with you, and to not understand what the treatment is supposed to do. You do not know how the human body works, your doctor does. Do what he says, *and understand why you are doing it!*

Many patients fail because they lack knowledge of very simple and commonsense concepts. They wind up receiving only partial treatment for conditions that need full treatment, or temporary for those that require permanent. *There is a definite and fundamental difference between the lack, or disappearance, of symptoms, and healing!* If you are going to treat your symptoms only, and not the underlying diseases, at least you should be aware of what you are doing. One example of this is stomach problems, be it simple esophagitis (heartburn), gastritis (inflamed stomach), or an ulcer. The burning, pain, or discomfort will likely disappear quickly from the treatment your doctor prescribes, perhaps in a few days or less. If you stop the treatment now, you are treating the symptom, not the disease. The inflamed tissues inside you can take as long as a month to heal. Many patients turn their acute problem into a chronic one. They forever chase their symptoms, dieting and taking medication only when they feel discomfort. Their insides never heal, are chronically inflamed, and periodically worsen slightly to cause symptoms.

There is another problem you may encounter if you do not follow your doctor's advice. If you come back to him with the same complaints, do not expect a similar degree of interest on his part. And if you lie to him about what you have done, be prepared to undergo a lot of costly and uncomfortable tests for probably no reason.

If you want to be a successful patient, you must understand what you are being treated for, what the treatment is supposed to do, and how long it is supposed to continue. Nowhere is there a greater incidence of failure than in the taking of medication. That topic will be discussed in another chapter.

In connection with your visit, you have probably been exposed to some medical terminology. Medical words are a frequent source of humor to a lot of patients. The terms all seem so complex and incomprehensible. It is not really all that complicated, however. Most medical terms are simply various combinations of relatively few prefixes and suffixes. One element of the word will identify the part of the body involved, and another element will state what is wrong with it. There are, of course, many exceptions. We are the inheritors of a large legacy of medical nomenclature from the past. Unfortunately, the lack of knowledge about disease processes led to inappropriate terms, and many of them are still in use. For those of you who are interested, I have listed some of the more common prefixes and suffixes, then put a few together to show you how they work.

PREFIXES

a- or an-	meaning without
arterio-	referring to arteries
arthr-	referring to joints
broncho-	referring to the bronchi
cholecyst-	referring to the gall bladder
col-	referring to the colon or large intestine
cyst-	referring to the urinary bladder
duoden-	referring to the duodenum
dys-	meaning abnormal, or discomfort with
endo-	referring to inside the body
esophaga-	referring to the esophagus
gastr-	referring to the stomach
glyc-	referring to sugar
hem-	referring to the blood
hepat-	referring to the liver
hyper-	more active, increased in quantity or function
hypo-	less active, decreased in quantity or function

leuk-	referring most commonly to white blood cells
lymph-	referring to a certain type of white blood cells or the glands where they are produced
myo-	referring to muscle
myocard-	referring to heart muscle
nephr-	referring to the kidneys
neur-	referring to nerves or the nervous system
osteo-	referring to bone
phleb-	referring to veins
pleur-	referring to the pleura, the lining of the lungs
pneumo-	referring to the lungs
prosta-	referring to the prostate
stoma-	referring to the mouth
thrombo-	referring to a blood clot

SUFFIXES

-algia	pain
-centesis	the removal of fluid
-cyte	a cell
-ectomy	removal
-emia	in the blood
-ism	a condition
-itis	inflammation or infection
-lithiasis	having a stone
-megaly	enlargement
-oma	a tumor (by itself does not signify whether benign or malignant)
-opathy	diseased
-oscopy	looking into with an instrument
-osis	having the condition
-ostomy	leaving a permanent or semipermanent opening
-otomy	opening it up
-paresis	weakness
-plegia	paralysis
-uria	having to do with urine

Now let us put some of them together and see what we get. I will leave a space between the prefix and the suffix. When you read the word, ignore the space.

TERMS

col ostomy	a permanent or semipermanent opening from the colon or large intestine for stool to empty through
cyst itis	a bladder infection
dys uria	painful urination
gastr oscopy	looking into the stomach with an instrument
hem arthr osis	having blood in a joint
hypo glyc emia	less than normal sugar in the blood
myocard opathy	a disease of the heart muscle
nephr ectomy	the removal of a kidney
neur algia	pain from a nerve
phleb otomy	opening a vein (what is done when you give blood for tests)

Sometimes, even chemical symbols of elements are used in medical words, such as hyperkalemia: hyper- (more than normal), K (chemical symbol for potassium), -emia (in the blood). Another such example is hyponatremia: hypo- (less than normal), Na (chemical symbol for sodium), -emia (in the blood).

Sometimes two words that seem almost the same actually describe two closely related but different conditions. For example: thrombophlebitis: thrombo- (there is a clot), phleb (in a vein), -itis (the vein is inflamed). Then there is phlebothrombosis: phlebo- (in a vein), thromb (a clot), -osis (exists). As you can see, the first word ended in *itis*, the second did not; there is no inflammation in this second condition.

These examples are, of course, only a few. As other medical words are used, I will also describe them where appropriate.

CHAPTER 7

TESTS

It is quite likely that your visit to the doctor will involve some kinds of medical tests. These may include a urinalysis, a series of blood tests, an electrocardiogram, a chest X-ray, or some other kind of diagnostic procedure. We live in a medical era of tests, all kinds of tests ranging from the myriad of available blood tests through various kinds of X-rays, sonograms, scans, endoscopies, and electrocardiograms. Medical tests are often critically important to either the establishment of a diagnosis or to the following of a patient's condition. Most patients do not realize that one very important reason for routine tests is the establishment of what physicians call a base line. This is simply the confirmation that everything is normal at that time, so that if anything in the future becomes abnormal, there will be some knowledge as to how long the condition has existed. This concept applies to blood tests, chest X-rays, and electrocardiograms.

As stated above, medical tests are extremely important, but they all have their limitations, far more limitations than patients realize. The fundamental question that should be in the mind of a patient, and should be asked, is: "How reliable is this test in determining what is wrong with me, or that I am healthy?" It has been my experience that most people have a totally unrealistic expectation of the answer to that question, of exactly what kind of information can be gained from medical tests.

This question of reliability in determining the presence or absence of disease is dependent upon two critical qualities of every test, *sensitivity* and *specificity*.

Before discussing what is meant by the sensitivity and specificity of tests in general, there is one other, less important, factor in this concept of test reliability: mistakes. Blood tests can be subject to errors that begin with the patient and end with the printing of the results in the laboratory. Many blood tests are dependent upon when the patient last ate, and it is surprising how many people forget a recent snack. Some tests require blood samples that are not allowed to clot, others on blood that has clotted. Tubes containing anticoagulants (to prevent clotting) may be faulty; sometimes the blood clots a little anyway. Sometimes the taking of the blood from the patient causes some of the red blood cells to break apart. This will make some of the determinations erroneous. Despite frequent checks on analytical machines and equipment, sometimes they do not work properly. Sometimes doctors, nurses, or technicians mislabel specimens, and results are reported for the wrong patient. It is true that none of these things should happen, but they do, and will, because everything ultimately is dependent upon us imperfect humans. Mistakes such as those described above are usually obvious, and customary medical routine calls for repeated determinations to confirm initial results. Mistakes can be made in other kinds of tests such as X-rays, sonograms, scans, etc. Sometimes the equipment is faulty, or a technician misses taking the right shots. Occasionally the radiologist reading the final product may miss seeing something that is there but very small. Most patients will understand that mistakes can happen, that abnormal findings have to be repeated. They do not realize, however, that mistakes such as outlined above are certainly the *least* important factor in the question of a test's reliability to detect illness or confirm health. So let us examine these concepts of innate sensitivity and specificity.

Sensitivity refers to how much disease must be present before a test will detect it. It should be obvious to all that no test is totally sensitive. No test can reveal when the first microscopic cell becomes malignant. No test can detect when the first microscopic deposits of fat appear in the wall of an artery. Some tests are fairly sensitive to the presence of disease. A very small amount of blood in a stool can be detected by chemically testing the feces for blood. White blood cells quickly appear in the urine when there is a urinary tract infection, and they are easily found. A Pap smear can reveal malignant changes in cells even before a true cancer develops. Other tests, many other tests, are relatively insensitive. Cancers of the lung have to be quite sizable, and have usually already spread, by the time they can be seen on a chest X-ray. Osteoporosis must be well advanced before there are any changes in a bone X-ray. Deterioration of kidney function must be quite advanced before the routine blood tests that check on that will become abnormal. Scans and sonograms cannot detect small masses or slight abnormalities in organs. A liver, for example, can be riddled with cancer that has spread from elsewhere, yet scans and sonograms of the liver will initially be normal. An upper G.I. series is a common test done to look for an ulcer, yet as many as one out of three ulcers cannot be seen this way.

There are three fundamental points to be understood from the above. The first is that when a test reveals an abnormality, the result is "probably" correct. The second is that when most tests are negative (that is to say, normal), they mean nothing at all. With some exceptions, normal tests simply cannot reliably rule out the presence of disease. The third point is that because of this lack of sensitivity, tests may have to be repeated when a disease or condition is seriously suspected. There have been numerous occasions when a patient will reply to my suggestion that a test be done: "But I had that test done two years ago!" How far removed from reality is his thinking when I would have insisted it be repeated even if done a month ago! This occasional necessity to repeat tests done fairly recently is part and parcel of their inherent lack of sensitivity. If a physician suspects something, if the symptoms persist, the tests must be repeated. Possibly the time interval will have allowed the condition to become detectable. I recall one elderly gentleman suffering from recurrent infections of a kidney. The urologist on the case and I could not keep him free of fever for more than a few weeks at a time. We did all the available tests, X-rays, sonograms, scans, repeatedly, and it was not until the fourth CAT scan that a tumor was detected. If your doctor believes that repeated tests are indicated for persistent symptoms, do not argue with him. But remember, also, that most diseases will manifest themselves in several completely different ways, and if your doctor is convinced there is nothing wrong and feels further testing is not indicated, do not argue with that either. Of course this is predicated on the assumption that he knows what he is doing.

Specificity is the other quality of a test you should understand. This concept revolves around the question of exactly how much information an abnormal laboratory result will yield, its implication. Some tests may provide your doctor with a diagnosis of a specific disease. An electrocardiogram can reveal a heart attack and its location. Blood tests can diagnose hepatitis, and what kind. An upper G.I. series can reveal a duodenal ulcer. Other tests may only be able to indicate that something is wrong with a system or organ, that any one of a few different conditions may be present. With some tests, abnormalities can be the result of many dozens of different diseases. When this happens, other tests are needed to track down the problem. A blood test that indicates a problem with kidney function, or that a patient is anemic, will probably not even begin to tell the doctor the nature of the disease process that is causing the problem. A sonogram or scan that reveals an enlarged liver or an enlarged spleen will seldom or rarely tell the physician *why* it is enlarged. The finding of a high white count alone does not tell the doctor why it is high. A differential count to learn which kind of white blood cell is elevated can tell him, for example, that either a viral or bacterial infection is present, but it still does not tell him the specifics, nor where the infection is. If your doctor tells you something is wrong and further tests are needed, you are certainly entitled to ask the nature of the problem. If you think he is being evasive, it is probably because he just cannot answer because of the test's lack of specificity. Do what he says, and remember that no matter how many times you ask, he cannot tell you what he does not know.

Undoubtedly the most common test done on a patient is a urinalysis. There are two parts to a really complete urinalysis, the chemical testing and the microscopic examination. Urine is usually chemically tested for sugar, blood, and protein, although there are other chemicals that are also often tested for. If blood or protein is present, the urine should also be examined microscopically. This yields additional information. The finding of red blood cells will confirm that blood is indeed present instead of free hemoglobin. The finding of large numbers of white blood cells will indicate an infection. Various kinds of microscopic casts may be found, which can indicate kidney diseases. Crystals seen in the urine can indicate what kind of kidney stone a patient is suffering from. This is by no means a complete list of what can be found by examining the urine. One note for women. When you are collecting a urine specimen in a cup, do what you can to avoid contaminating it with vaginal secretions. It is best to wipe the area with a wet paper towel, then keep the vaginal lips separated while passing the urine.

Tests done on blood are among the most common performed. All married people have had at least one blood test, to determine if they have syphilis. How many different kinds of tests can be done on blood? I have never counted, but the number is probably in the hundreds. I do a routine series of approximately thirty different blood tests on new patients and those coming to see me for a periodic checkup. Some of these, I admit, are of marginal value, but most are very important. Some physicans may do fewer, some more, but it is certainly true that no checkup can be complete without a basic blood survey to learn things about a patient that simply cannot be learned any other way.

I believe patients should have some idea of what kinds of fairly common tests exist, what they measure and mean, and which ones are being done on their blood. Most series of blood tests are generally thought of as including a CBC and blood chemistries, the latter an all-inclusive term for most things of a chemical nature measured in the blood. The following section contains a brief description of blood tests that are commonly part of a routine physical examination.

A CBC stands for complete blood count. This measures the numbers and kinds of white blood cells. It also measures the amount of red blood cells, to determine whether the patient is anemic. Two other tests, the hemoglobin and hematocrit, also determine the presence and severity of anemia. They are much more accurate than a simple count of the red blood cells. The hemoglobin is a chemical measurement of the hemoglobin content of those red blood cells. The hematocrit is simply a measurement of what percentage of your whole blood is red blood cells.

A BUN and electrolytes is a common grouping of blood chemistries. The BUN is a measure of kidney function, but it is not very sensitive. A great deal of kidney function must be lost before the test becomes abnormal. Electrolytes are the sodium, potassium, chloride, and bicarbonate in your blood. They are of importance in patients taking diuretics (water pills), patients receiving intravenous fluids in a hospital, and those seriously ill.

There is a grouping of tests commonly called liver chemistries. These include tests called SGPT, SGOT, LDH, Alk. Phos., and bilirubin. The term *liver chemistries* is somewhat misleading since diseases other than those affecting the liver will cause most to be abnormal. The capital letters are abreviations of enzymes found in the blood. These enzymes are made, by and large, inside various cells, and are released into the blood when those cells die or are injured by disease. The SGOT and LDH, among others, also become elevated in a heart attack, and the Alk. Phos. is increased in some bone diseases.

The albumin and globulin are the two main categories of proteins in the blood. The albumin becomes low when a patient is malnourished, particularly in the elderly, or when a great deal of protein is being lost in the urine. Very low quantities of albumin can be one cause of retention of fluid and swelling of tissues. The globulins are the kinds of proteins that include antibodies, the chemicals made by the body to kill foreign cells or microorganisms, and to neutralize foreign chemicals. When globulins are found to be elevated, further tests, an electrophoresis and possibly others, must be done. This tells your doctor whether many different globulins are elevated—as is the case with rheumatoid arthritis, chronic infectious or inflammatory diseases, and cirrhosis of the liver, as some examples—or whether the elevation is due to a malignant condition of the cells that make the globulins.

The calcium and the phosphorous are two tests that check for any condition causing the calcium concentration in the blood to be abnormal. Osteoporosis most definitely does *not* affect this test. It should be done as part of a routine physical examination mainly to detect unsuspected parathyroid adenomas. These are very tiny, usually benign, tumors in the neck that secrete too much of a hormone that controls the blood calcium level. Elevated calcium levels can cause significant damage to the body and the mind, without anyone suspecting that anything is amiss. I usually find one unsuspected case about every two years, and the change in patients thought to have a problem with a stubborn ulcer, or early senility, can be dramatic when the benign tumor is removed. Anyone with these problems or recurrent calcium kidney stones should certainly be sure that this is checked.

There are several tests that measure the amount of thyroid hormone in the blood, and these also should be checked periodically. It is not at all unusual to find mildly underactive thyroid glands in patients who basically seem to be healthy. This is especially true in the elderly where mild symptoms of hypothyroidism (an underactive thyroid gland) can be attributed to old age. I have on occasion even found slightly over-active thyroid glands (hyperthyroidism) in patients that I did not suspect to have the condition. Much more information about these conditions will be found in the chapter dealing with the thyroid.

Tests to determine the blood levels of lipids (fats) are important in all ages, but contrary to what seems to be the popular notion, the younger the patient, the more important it is. These tests include the cholesterol, triglycerides, and others, all of which seem to have some connection with rapid progression of hardening of the arteries. That condition is discussed in Chapter 13.

The above is certainly not an exhaustive list of blood tests, nor even those most commonly done. Many physicians routinely check their patients for syphilis. Many other kinds of tests are done on patients with specific problems. Patients about to undergo surgery usually routinely have a test called a prothrombin time (PT) and a partial thromboplastin time (PTT) done. These check on the ability of the blood to clot normally. A platelet count is also usually done. Clotting and platelets are discussed in the chapter dealing with the blood. Typing of red blood cells in preparation for a transfusion, and cross-checking that they are compatible with the potential recipient, are other tests done prior to surgery.

A blood test called a sedimentation rate is often done by physicians. This test has great sensitivity to a wide variety of medical problems, specificity therefore being completely absent. It can tell a physician if one of many types of disease processes is present, and is often used to follow the course of diseases like rheumatoid arthritis.

All of the above tests are done on venous blood. If you are not certain of the difference between veins and arteries, it is spelled out in Chapter 13. There are some tests done on arterial blood. They measure the actual amount of oxygen, carbon dioxide, and acidity in your blood and under certain circumstances are very important. They are commonly called arterial blood gases.

There are, of course, many tests that do not involve analyzing the blood. One of the more common of these is the electrocardiogram (EKG or ECG). It has been around a long time, but few patients seem to understand what information it yields, or its limitations. An electrocardiogram measures the electric current generated by the heart muscle during its contraction and relaxation, more specifically its depolarization and repolarization. Changes in this current can reveal evidence of areas of the heart that are relatively deprived of blood, areas that have died or been damaged from old heart attacks, and evidence of enlargement or excessive strain. The EKG will also reveal abnormalities of the heart's rhythm, if it is beating too fast or too slow, and why. *But it can only reveal what is happening during the time it is being taken*. Patients will often complain about having experienced palpitations some time in the past, then wonder why the EKG does not reveal what the problem is. The same thing holds true for angina. The EKG is very often normal if the patient is not experiencing symptoms while it is being taken. The test also cannot predict the future. The stories about people dropping dead from a heart attack immediately after a normal EKG are only surprising to those who do not understand its limitations. Nevertheless, the EKG is an important and useful test. It can reveal problems otherwise undetectable, and changes do provide some information as to a patient's cardiac condition. Alternate methods of having electrocardiograms are discussed in Chapter 14.

X-rays form a large portion of medical tests. We will review those most commonly done.

A chest X-ray is undoubtedly the most common X-ray procedure, but most patients are unaware of its rather severe limitations, and I believe it is overused. It is relatively insensitive. In cases such as tumors or emphysema, a great deal of disease must be present before it will be seen. In the past it became a routine test mainly because of the prevalence of tuberculosis. With much less of that disease around, I do not think it is so necessary as a matter of routine. Many patients with pneumonia will have multiple chest X-rays to follow its course. Again, changes in the chest X-ray lag far behind the actual improvement in the patient, and it is of limited value except in unusual cases.

Bones are often X-rayed after some form of trauma. Broken bones can be seen well, and immediately, but a minute crack in a bone may not become visible for some time after it occurs.

Many X-rays are done with contrast material. Contrast material is something that will show up on the X-ray. Barium is swallowed for an upper G.I. series to show the esophagus, stomach, and some of the small intestine, and it is used for an enema to show the large intestine (colon). Other kinds of contrast material are injected. They can reveal the kidneys and urinary tract in an intravenous pyelogram (IVP), arteries in an arteriogram (also called angiogram), and veins in a venogram, among many others.

X-ray examinations of the stomach and intestines usually consist of an upper G.I. series and barium enema. Remember, it is only the barium that can be seen. The absence of the material where it should be, or its presence where it should not be, leads to an inference as to what is actually there. Abnormalities in these tests are often confirmed by either a gastroscopy or colonoscopy (see endoscopies below).

An intravenous pyelogram is a common test to see the kidneys, the tubes that carry the urine to the bladder, and the bladder itself. It is a fairly sensitive test to detect physical abnormalities and can help to evaluate kidney function.

An arteriogram gives your doctor a look at your arteries. This test can be done to check almost any major artery when a blockage is suspected. It is fairly accurate in detecting significant problems.

A sonogram has nothing to do with X-rays at all. The machinery produces sound waves that enter your body and echo back to a receiver. Since tissues of different densities reflect sound waves differently, a picture can be made of the returning echoes. Sonograms vary in their reliability and sensitivity depending upon what area of the body is being examined. Negative findings may mean nothing, especially if your doctor really suspects something.

A great many tests are called scans. There are thyroid, liver, brain, bone, heart, and CAT scans, among others. They are important and useful tests, but not as reliable in detecting disease and differentiating between diseases as we would like, and as most patients suppose. I recently hospitalized a patient with a very high persistent fever, a very slight pain in the right side of her back, and evidence of a urinary tract infection. She only partially responded to antibiotic therapy. A complete evaluation of her urinary tract revealed nothing, and that included sonograms and CAT scans. Both the urologist and I felt strongly that we were missing something, but the patient ultimately improved and was discharged. A few months later her symptoms reappeared. This time the tests revealed an abscess next to her right kidney. It had certainly been there earlier, but it was undetectable.

The term *endoscopy* means looking into the body with an instrument. There are many different kinds of endoscopies, all named according to what part of the body is being looked into. These are among the most reliable, sensitive, and specific tests available. With modern equipment the endoscopist can actually see within the body, visualize the disease, and take biopsies for pathologic examination. There is, however, a price to be paid for this increased sensitivity and specificity. They are more formidable tests. There is more discomfort, more chance for complications, and sometimes anesthesia is required. Let your doctor decide if an endoscopy is an appropriate test for you.

A gastroscopy involves looking at the esophagus, stomach, and the beginning of the small intestine, the duodenum.

There are three names for endoscopy done through the rear, the anus. A proctoscopy visualizes the rectum, the last several inches of the large intestine. A sigmoidoscopy includes the last couple of feet of the large intestine. A colonoscopy allows visualization of the entire large intestine.

A cystoscopy is done by a urologist. It allows him to see the urinary bladder and whether an enlarged prostate is causing obstruction. Other procedures can be done during a cystoscopy. The prostate can be shaved away to relieve the obstruction, bladder stones and tumors removed, or tiny tubes can be placed in the ureters, the ducts coming from the kidneys, to either bypass an obstruction there or to inject contrast material to get a better X-ray of them.

Gynecologists will often do a culdoscopy through the vagina. This allows them a direct look at the ovaries and Fallopian tubes.

A bronchoscopy allows visualization of the windpipe, the trachea, and the bronchi. It can be done with a rigid tube that allows easier biopsy of any mass, or with a flexible instrument that can penetrate more deeply into smaller bronchi.

A laparoscopy involves a direct look into the abdominal cavity. This is often a procedure of choice instead of formal surgery to explore the abdomen.

These are not all the endoscopic procedures available, but they are the most common. Again, in most cases an endoscopy will provide the most accurate information.

The test called a "culture" seems to be confusing to many patients. This test is done when an infection is either suspected or confirmed. It will tell your doctor whether any microorganisms (germs) are present, which ones they are, and what antibiotic will be most effective in eliminating them. In order to really understand about cultures you have to have some understanding about infections. That subject is discussed in Chapter 20.

A culture is done by putting the material to be tested for the presence of microorganisms onto gelatinlike substances and into various culture solutions. These media contain nutrients designed to encourage the growth of all or certain kinds of bacteria. The test is most commonly done on urine, sputum, pus, and blood, although many other materials such as stool and spinal fluid are also sometimes cultured. Bacteria grow very fast, and if present will either make a solution cloudy with their numbers or form tiny mounds on the gelatin media. The bacteria are then tested further to determine exactly which kind they are and which antibiotics will be most effective in killing them.

Like all tests, cultures are not perfect. Sometimes an infection is present but the organism cannot be found. Sometimes it is an uncommon kind of germ that will not grow in the media.

Cultures are not necessary in all infections. It depends on the site and seriousness of the infection. Your doctor can very often make an educated guess as to what organism is present and what antibiotic will kill it and be right ninety-nine percent of the time. Two examples of this would be a boil, which is almost always caused by staphylococcus, and a bladder infection in an otherwise healthy female, which is usually caused by one of a few microorganisms. Cultures do become a necessity when the infection is either unusual, recurrent, or very serious.

Another common kind of test is the biopsy. Often, in order for your doctor to know the nature of a mass or abnormal fluid in your body, a piece or sample will be taken for a pathologist to look at. These are very important tests, and pathologists often send the material to other pathologists for second opinions.

If there is one concept you should gain from all the above, it is that medical tests vary greatly in both what information they can yield, and the degree of discomfort and risk involved in doing them. A physician will quite naturally want to do the least complicated ones first, others only if they are indicated. This will depend upon the nature and degree of your symptoms. Beware the M.D. who jumps to do everything immediately as much as the one who does nothing.

I must repeat a point I have emphasized before. Despite the hundreds of different tests that can be done on blood, and despite the sophisticated X-rays, sonograms, and scanning equipment, *a diagnosis is most commonly arrived at from your history and physical examination. The tests are done to confirm what your doctor suspects.* In my opinion, it will be that way for the foreseeable future. Medicine remains, today, one quarter science and three quarters art.

Are medical tests being done unnecessarily, to any substantial degree? Most emphatically yes! *And at a truly enormous expense.* I believe that a very substantial portion of the high total cost of medicine is due to this. We all should have some concern about the costs of medical care, whether we pay for it directly or indirectly through third parties or taxes. Cost has to be one of the determining factors in what we elect to do routinely. There are several reasons for this overtesting, and the primary ones include the malpractice situaton and contemporary medical economic policies.

There is what I call the "We'd better get a . . ." complex among physicians. Those very words are thought, and said, every day by the practicing medical community. They have little, if anything, to do with medical care. They mean that physicians are under intense pressure to do all possible tests for every complaint on every patient. Many physicians reason as follows: You have to cover your tracks, because you never know when some lawyer is going to accusingly ask you in court why you did not do one specific test or another. Many, if not most, physicians reflexively order expensive diagnostic procedures for minimal symptoms without first attempting a trial of treatment based upon their clinical diagnoses, diagnoses that in most cases are as accurate, or more accurate, than those derived from X-rays, scans, etc.

Let us consider a hypothetical case of a man in his forties going to see a doctor because of a pain in the pit of his abdomen. The doctor believes the patient has an ulcer and prescribes appropriate treatment and medication. The cost so far can range from, say, $35 to $150 depending upon the physician and whether it is a first visit or not. Perhaps the physician also did an electrocardiogram and blood tests, maybe another $75 or so. We have then a total top cost of about $225, and as little as $35. Now comes the waste. Instead of treating the patient on the basis of his clinical diagnosis, instead of waiting a few days to see if the patient improves, the doctor orders an upper G.I. series and an abdominal sonogram, because you never know who is going to sue you. I mean, it is *possible* that there is something else wrong with the patient. Those two tests, at a local radiologist, cost $375. If the doctor has been sued a couple of times, he will probably also want a barium enema. Add on another $200. If the doctor has actually been involved in a trial, if he has been in court, he will also want a CAT scan for $375, and undoubtedly will send the patient to a gastroenterologist for a gastroscopy. Add on another $500 or more. The malpractice situation has converted a $35 to $225 illness into one costing well over $1500. Do not think this is at all unusual. It is an all-pervasive way of thinking, and it goes on every day, in every office, in every hospital, with almost every patient. And to top it all, if the doctor really knows what he is doing, he does not really care what all those tests show! He is going to treat the patient according to his clinical diagnosis, and be right ninety-nine percent of the time! And if he is wrong, he will know in a few days anyway because the patient will not get better! And if the patient does have something else, like a tumor of the pancreas or stomach for example, the few days' delay in making the diagnosis will have meant nothing at all to the patient's prognosis!

There are the beginnings of some attempts to control this. For example, in some hospitals only neurologists and neurosurgeons can order CAT scans of the brain. The result is only the added cost of the specialist's consultation! Physicians reflexively call in a neurologist for *any* neurologic problem, and neurologists *always* order CAT scans of the brain. They get sued also. There may one day be even stronger attempts to regulate and limit diagnostic procedures, but they will be doomed to failure. The physician fears the malpractice attorney far more than he does the insurance company or government bureaucrat.

A substantial part of the answer to the high cost of medicine is simply to encourage a shift in medical thinking, away from immediate thousand-dollar diagnostic precedures to, in most cases, a trial of therapy based on clinical diagnoses. The time to do the tests is when the patient fails to respond as expected. Serious conditions and diseases are, by and large, not significantly worsened by a short delay in diagnosis if the physician attempts a reasonable period of therapy for an erroneous diagnosis.

The other reason for the plethora of unnecessary diagnostic testing is something I have mentioned earlier. Procedures and tests pay much better than time spent with the patient. A fifteen-minute procedure can bring in three to ten times the amount of dollars that spending a half hour taking a careful history will. Physicians are only human; they will certainly bend and conform to the economic realities. It is unfortunate. A physician's time is so much more valuable and rewarding.

CHAPTER 8

MEDICATION

Nowhere do people fail as patients more than in the taking of prescribed medication. In my experience, most of the time it is due to ignorance of two very simple and fundamental concepts of medicinal therapy.

The first concept is that some medications are meant to be taken for a *limited* period of time, some on an *as-needed* basis, and some *indefinitely*, forever.

Antibiotics for an infection are a good example of the first kind, as are antispasmodics for cramps due to an intestinal virus, and antacids and other medication for an acute ulcer problem. These medications either "cure" the condition, or are taken until the condition goes away.

The second kind of medication is for problems that are recurrent, but not continual. Aspirin for a headache, antispasmodics for a spastic colon, some asthma medication, and tranquilizers for recurrent anxiety, are examples of these. You take the medication whenever you need it.

Many medications, however, are taken for a condition that is chronic and persistent, such as hypertension, hardening of the arteries, diabetes, or excessively high uric acid levels predisposing to gout and kidney disease. *In these instances the medication is "controlling" a condition, not "curing" it. There is no lasting beneficial effect once it is stopped!* Many times I have placed a patient with diabetes or hypertension on medication only to hear months or years later that they had stopped their medication after having found that their sugar was normal, or that their pressure was normal when checked in a mall or a department store. The medication leaves their bodies within a day or two usually, and from that point on they again have high blood sugar or high blood pressure.

It is very important for you to know how long you should take any prescribed medication. If you are not certain, ask your doctor. Should you just finish the bottle? Or take it as needed? Or take it indefinitely?

The second concept that patients should understand is that *some medications are given for relief of symptoms only. They are not important to, and do not improve, your general health or life expectancy.* Examples include arthritis pills, some heart medication, and pain medication. Other medications, however, *do improve your health, prevent severe medical problems or complications, and prolong your life.* I believe it is very important that every patient knows these facts about their medications. If you decide you do not like taking pills anymore, at least you should be aware of the possible consequences.

Another common source of confusion over taking medications is the timing. Not everyone understands what two times a day or three times a day means. Others are unreasonably concerned over taking medications together, and complicate their lives needlessly by waiting an hour between taking pills that could all be taken together.

Once a day means in the morning unless otherwise specified. Twice a day means approximately twelve hours apart, ten to fourteen hours is fine. Three times a day means in the morning, at night, and about half way between. Four times a day means at mealtimes and before bed. If you are not certain when you should take your pills, do not hesitate to ask your doctor or pharmacist. It is their responsibility to inform you.

Under most circumstances, if you are taking more than one medication at the same time, they can be taken together. It is done that way in hospitals. There is no need, with most medication, to allow a time interval. Again, if you are concerned or unsure, ask!

All patients taking medication should know the names, both brand and generic, of the pills they are taking, and the dosage strength. If this cannot be remembered, they should write it down on paper and keep it in their wallet. Patients should also know what "kind" of medicine they are taking, the purpose of it, what it is supposed to do. There is nothing to be gained by ignorance. I will never forget the woman who first came to my office complaining of very severe weakness. I mean she was so weak she could barely stand! She brought along her pills that she took every day, six bottles of them. Every bottle had a different name on it, but *all six were diuretics!* There were two different generic names, and four different brand names, of two kinds of water pills! The woman was so weak because she was greatly overdosed with diuretics and severely depleted in sodium and potassium. All the pills had been prescribed by the same doctor over a period of time. It was his fault that he never bothered to find out if she was still taking old prescriptions, but the potentially catastrophic problem could have been avoided if the patient had made the slightest inquiry into what "kind" of medication each prescription was. You, as a patient, must assume the ultimate responsibility for your health. You must be the final safety check. No doctor is God, not one is infallible, not one never makes a mistake.

While we're on the subject of medication, let's devote a little time to the discussion and understanding of side effects. The term *side effect* refers to any unwanted effect of a medication. Most side effects can be thought of as belonging to one of the following categories: 1, allergic in nature; 2, fairly common complications that are usually not too serious; or 3, idiosyncratic reactions.

An allergic reaction to a medication is only one kind of side effect. The body's immune system, sensing that the medication, or the medication attached to a protein in the blood, is foreign to the body, reacts to it as if it were a foreign germ, and produces antibodies that attach to the medication. This causes the release of histamine and other chemicals, which results in what we see and feel as an allergic reaction. When the medication is taken orally, by mouth, the absorption into the blood is relatively slow, and the most common manifestation is itchy hives, raised red weals. There is a much greater danger when the medication is given by injection. The sudden flood into the blood can cause a very serious reaction that, in some cases, can result in death. All doctors, of course, are very aware of that possibility, and there is medication that can quickly stop the allergic reaction.

There are other kinds of allergic reactions that involve inflammation of the skin instead of hives. These can be particularly severe, especially if the medication is still taken after the reaction begins.

It is important to understand that you *become* allergic to a medication, as a result of taking it. Commonly, you have to take it many times, or many, many times, or for a relatively long period of time, before your body either begins to develop antibodies, or develops enough of them for you to be aware of an allergic reaction. So when your doctor tells you that you are having an allergic reaction, do not say: "But I've taken that before without any problem!" He already knows that.

There are many medications that quite commonly, or even usually, cause nonallergic side effects. Arthritis or anti-inflammatory medication often produces inflammation of the stomach, or even an ulcer. Some high blood pressure medication can cause drowsiness, lethargy, or even impotence. Codeine, when first taken, commonly causes nausea, as do some forms of the antibiotic erythromycin. Antacids can cause diarrhea. *None of these are allergies.* Sometimes these side effects go away with continued use. Sometimes measures can be taken to prevent or eliminate them. Sometimes the medication has to be discontinued.

"Idiosyncratic side effects" refers to very rare reactions to medications, occuring perhaps in only one of hundreds of thousands, or even millions, of individuals who take them. These reactions can most commonly affect the blood, the bone marrow where blood cells are made, or the liver. Most of the time they are reversible, meaning that the problem goes away when the medication is stopped. Sometimes, rarely, these reactions can be fatal. *This is an important reason to have periodic checkups and blood tests when you are taking medication.*

I certainly cannot discuss the specifics of all kinds of medications in this book, but I will discuss those that are commonly prescribed and have caused the most confusion among my patients.

Water pills, or diuretics, are given for one of two purposes, either to rid the body of excess water, or to lower the blood pressure by doing the same thing. There are many different kinds, and dozens of brands, of diuretics, differing mainly in potency and duration of action, but they all have the same end effect, to increase the elimination or excretion of sodium (salt) through the kidneys. By and large, where the sodium goes, so goes the water, so by increasing the elimination of sodium in the urine, more water is passed. Diuretics do *not* have any effect on the urinary bladder, and they only *may* make you urinate more often. Many times I have heard from a patient with a degree of prostatic obstruction or urethral stenosis, both of which can make you urinate frequently, that "I don't need a water pill. I urinate a lot!" *Do not confuse the "passing" of urine with the "production" of urine.* Patients who habitually take a diuretic for high blood pressure will undergo a loss of sodium and water from the body during the first few days or weeks that they take the medication, but this loss is self-limited. If they remain on a low salt intake, an equilibrium will be reached and there will be no significant difference in their urination.

Most diuretics also cause the kidneys to excrete more potassium. Potassium is something we need, and most patients taking a diuretic on an ongoing basis will need potassium replacement. *Drinking orange juice or eating bananas can help, but seldom provide enough potassium to make up for what is lost in the urine.*

A word here about taking diuretics as an adjunct to dieting to lose weight. *Diuretics have no effect on fat!* If you are otherwise healthy, you will lose several pounds of water by taking a water pill. If you take it daily for ten years, there will still only be the loss of those first original few pounds. When you stop it, the weight will be regained within twenty-four to forty-eight hours. It hardly pays to take a potent medication just to partially dehydrate yourself, to purposefully fool yourself with a scale reading.

There are many different brands and kinds of blood pressure medication, and they work in many different ways. It would be too confusing to describe their various mechanisms of action. All I will say is that *they only work while in your body. They have no lasting effect once you stop taking them.* And I will say it again later.

Antibiotics are given to kill (or perhaps it is better to say "sicken") the bacteria causing an infection. There are many different kinds of antibiotics, and new ones keep appearing with almost confusing frequency. Some of them can be taken by mouth, others have to be given by injection either into a muscle or intravenously. Many times I have heard a patient say: "That antibiotic doesn't work on me," or "Is that antibiotic strong enough?" Those statements are kind of silly. Antibiotics are not medications for "you" in the sense that other medicines are. They only have an effect on certain germs. If they do have an effect on "you," it is probably an undesirable side effect. And there is really no such thing as "strength" when it comes to an antibiotic. Either the germ is sensitive to it, and the antibiotic will work, or the germ is resistant, and the antibiotic will do little or nothing. One more thing about antibiotics. They are *not* given to reduce fever. The fever goes down when the infection gets better, and that can take a few days.

Anti-inflammatory medications, otherwise known as arthritis pills, are many and varied. There is no great difference between them, although it is true that some will work better on some patients, and others are more effective in other patients. I believe it does pay to try a few. They basically all, however, have the same primary side effect, and that is to cause stomach inflammation. I often tell my patients to take antacids on a regular basis *before* they get their stomach symptoms. It is easier to prevent the stomach inflammation than to cure it, because once it begins you have to stop the anti-inflammatory medication.

There are three basic kinds of medication for angina, which are discussed on the chapter dealing with the heart. Understand that one of the most commonly used kind has very little, if anything, to do with your health. It does not make your heart better, or stronger, and it cannot stop a heart attack. It simply stops or prevents heart pain. The movie scene of the old man reaching in desperation for his bottle of pills, only to die before reaching it, is a total myth.

Pills for diabetes all work the same way. There will be very little difference in your blood sugar if you are taking the top dose of any of them. Their major differences are in their duration of action and possible side effects. There is more information about them in the chapter on diabetes.

Many patients shrink in horror from the mere mention of the word *cortisone*. It is understandable, but too often I have encountered an unreasonable total refusal to even consider taking it. It is true that prolonged use of significant doses of cortisone causes severe side effects. It is also true, however, that taking large doses for a short period of time, or small doses for a prolonged period of time, cause few, and controllable, side effects. The amount of cortisone that you get from a shot for bursitis, for example, is very minimal. So be cautious about taking cortisone, but do not reflexively refuse.

There are many medications given for the purpose of reducing the blood's potential to form clots. Using their generic names, these include heparin, warfarin, aspirin, and dipyrimadole. If the following is confusing to you, reread it after reading Chapter 11 on the blood, Chapter 13 on the vascular system, and Chapter 15 on the lungs.

Heparin interferes directly with clotting. It must be given by injection. Warfarin also interferes with clotting, but only by depleting the blood of chemicals necessary for a clot to form. It is an effective medication, but not quite as effective as heparin. Warfarin is commonly taken at home by patients who have had thrombophlebitis, a pulmonary embolus, certain kinds of strokes, or certain kinds of heart problems. Patients taking warfarin have to be tested periodically to measure how fast or slowly their blood is clotting. The PT test, mentioned earlier, serves as a guide for their doctor to know how much warfarin they need to take for their blood to clot in the proper amount of time.

Two more notes about warfarin. It does not "thin" your blood, as so many people mistakenly say. Secondly, there are many medications that will significantly either lessen or enhance its effectiveness. Your doctor, or doctors, should know if you either begin taking a new medication, or stop one that you have been taking.

Tranquilizers and sleeping pills are popular, and controversial, prescription items. There are only a few "classes" of these kinds of medications, but many different variations and brands within each class. The older kinds, especially of sleeping pills, were barbiturates. These, I believe, should be avoided because of their tendency to cause addiction. There is some potential for addiction in the newer ones also, but to a much lesser extent. I will have more to say on the use of these kinds of medications in a later chapter. I would like to say here that I see nothing wrong with their judicious use, that they are certainly not going to solve any of your problems, and that the more you use a sleeping pill, the less effective it will be.

The final kind of medication I would like to discuss is laxatives. They are overused by many, many people, and over a period of many years will cause damage to the large intestine, at least to the extent of creating dependency upon them. Do not take laxatives on a daily basis, if you have to take them at all. There is more on this subject in the chapter dealing with the gastrointestinal tract.

CHAPTER 9

THE HOSPITAL

A common question among patients is whether any given hospital is a "good" hospital. I have never quite fully understood the meaning of the term. I have frequently asked patients what they mean by that, but have never received a rational response. The following discussion is not meant to apply to patients who are being admitted to a hospital for a special type of procedure that may be done in only a few specialized institutions. It also would not apply to patients who are being admitted without a personal physician there to care for them.

As far as a patient is concerned, there are two basic kinds of hospitals, the large university-affiliated teaching hospital, and the usually smaller nonteaching hospital. The greatest difference between these types of hospitals is the presence or absence of a house staff, that is, interns and residents. The presence or absence of a house staff can make a difference in your care. The problem is that you do not know beforehand which way the difference will apply. Should an emergency arise, it may be helpful to have all those doctors around twenty-four hours a day. But on the other hand, hospitals without a house staff hire physicians who stay in the hospital twenty-four hours a day. You are more likely to receive a very thorough going-over with a house staff present, but then again, physicians in training have a strong tendency to overdo it when it comes to ordering tests. I have had patients in both types of institutions over the years, patients for whom I was their primary care physician, and patients I have seen in hematologic consultation. On the whole I have found it easier to care for my patients in the nonteaching type of institution. There are exceptions to this, but they are few. The factor that I see as making the biggest difference for me has been the lack of interference from a house staff with a lot of knowledge and little experience. I am sure many physicians will totally disagree with this opinion.

I see three factors that would affect you during a hospital stay. The first and foremost is the physician or physicians who are going to take care of you. There may be several doctors who see you during a hospital stay, but only one will have the ultimate responsibility for your care. That physician is generally the one who admits you to the hospital. If it is your regular physician, and he is going to call in others if necessary, then the rest of the doctors on the staff of the hospital should not be of any concern to you because your doctor will only use those who are up to snuff. Many patients seem to have a feeling that one hospital or another has better doctors, or that the large teaching hospital has all the professors. The truth is that most physicians are on the staff of many hospitals, and the professor at the university-affiliated teaching institution may be the same specialist who sees you at a little hospital a few miles away. As a matter of fact, he may pay more attention to you in the small hospital because he is not busy talking to the interns and residents. I admit many of my patients to a small hospital. The chest surgeon I use, for example, has been the chief of surgery at two university-affiliated teaching hospitals. Please do not think that I am saying that only the professors are the good doctors; that is certainly not the case. Remember, there are only two kinds of doctors, the ones who know what they are doing, and the ones who do not. If you have a primary care physician who has an interest in your well-being, he will only have competent physicians of at least equal ability see you in consultation should that be necessary.

The second factor is the nursing care you will receive. It is true that the quality of nursing care will vary from hospital to hospital, but it is far more likely that it will vary much more from floor to floor, and from shift to shift, within the same hospital. Nurses, like the rest of us, are only human. Some care and some do not. It is mostly a matter of drawing straws.

The final factor is the laboratory facilities. Here again there may be variation between hospitals, but the degree of difference for most routine types of tests is small.

I will tell you my fondest recollection of family concern over the quality of a hospital. An elderly patient of mine was brought to a local hospital suffering from both pneumonia and pulmonary edema (water in the lungs). He stopped breathing as he was brought to emergency room and went into convulsions. The emergency room staff cleared his airway, an anesthesiologist got a tube into his lungs, and they got him breathing again. Then he suddenly died, his heart stopped beating. Once again he was resuscitated, brought back to life. Several days later he was in much better condition, awake and alert, but he needed a tracheostomy, a very quick and simple surgical procedure. After all that had happened, the family wanted to know if the hospital was good enough for it to be done there!

In summation, the most important part of being in a hospital is the primary doctor who is going to be taking care of you. For ninety-nine percent of illnesses, it makes very little difference which kind of hospital you are in, as long as your doctor knows what he is doing.

CHAPTER 10

NUTRITION, VITAMINS, AND DIETING

There are recurrent outbreaks of nutrition consciousness in our society, one dietary vogue and fad after another becoming popular, then fading away. I will begin by saying that almost all of it is nonsense. That is not to say that I do not think good nutrition is important, it most definitely is, but the lengths to which some so-called experts go to describe good nutrition is farcical.

My comments here about vitamins and minerals will undoubtedly arouse the wrath of many people, but they mirror the opinion of most physicians not involved in some way with the "health" industry. My basic belief is as follows: The animals and vegetables that we consume are nutritious. If we choose a balanced variety of these foods, we will be well nourished, and will get our required quota of vitamins and minerals. Almost everything you hear and read about the value of supplemental vitamins and minerals has little or no foundation in fact. The industry preys upon the scientific naiveté of the public, citing scientific studies or principles that, for the most part, are probably not fraudulent, but are, for all intents and purposes, worthless. They typically take a kernel of medical and scientific truth, then expand it to such ridiculous proportions that the conclusions you inevitably draw have little to do with reality. The problem is that proponents of vitamins are not required to prove their value. If vitamins and minerals came under the same federal regulations as medications, the industry would probably close down overnight. Their claims as to the therapeutic benefits of their products are simply unsubstantiated by proper medical and scientific investigation.

My patients who have fallen for all the literature on the beneficial effects of this and that vitamin or mineral, and are thoroughly convinced of their efficacy, will often look at me with wonder and confusion. I can see the various thoughts on their faces. How can he be so closed minded? they wonder. How can he not believe all that scientific evidence? they wonder. How can he be so ignorant? The simple truth is that physicians cannot be sold the bill of goods that those less educated, and more gullible, have been. I have never seen a case of pellagra due to niacin deficiency, nor beriberi due to thiamin deficiency, nor scurvy due to a lack of vitamin C. Indeed, overeating is the far greater health problem in this country, not undernourishment.

What I see in my patients seems to be only part of a pervasive belief, despite the lack of scientific evidence, among a substantial segment of the population that favors the therapeutic claims of vitamin proponents in their disagreement with the medical "establishment." We are the benficiaries of a vast interconnected research network involving public and private corporations and universities, institutions and people who are doing first-rate work, the cutting edge of one aspect of medical research. These same people, with all their intense and complex research methods, cannot find evidence to support the great bulk of the therapeutic claims made by vitamin proponents. Yet, so many people take these documented findings and opinions on what vitamins and minerals can and cannot do with a grain of salt, as if there were some reason these researchers would want to hush up or minimize some therapeutic benefit. Indeed, some people are of the notion that there is some form of a conspiracy in the medical profession against vitamins and minerals, that we are set against them for one selfish reason or another. That is just simply nonsense. We base our opinions on medical evidence, and in our view, those ardent and loyal proponents of vitamins and minerals are excessively therapeutically naive.

Let us look at one blatant example of this. I have had patients tell me that the B vitamins are supposed to be good for "nerves." Significant nutritional deficiencies in some of the B vitamins do cause neuropathies, degeneration of real nerves, or even of the spinal cord. But to take that fact and transpose it to the term *nervous*, to think that vitamins have any significant effect on "anxiety," is appallingly ridiculous.

Another more recent example of this almost quackery is the calcium and osteoporosis business. The physiologic and biochemical facts are that calcium can do little, if anything at all, for osteoporosis. The problem in osteoporosis is the loss of the protein matrix of the bone, the internal structure to which calcium adheres. Once this support is lost, the calcium disappears and will not be replaced no matter how much calcium is consumed. One normally builds a wall by first putting up wood studs, then nailing sheetrock or plasterboard to it. In this comparison the studs are the protein matrix of bone and the plasterboard is the calcium. If the plasterboard falls off, you can nail on a new piece. If termites have eaten the studs, however, you cannot nail plasterboard to air! The term *fraud* is not far from mind when you have a representative of a major pharmaceutical firm come into your office, ask you to recommend his brand of calcium, and then sheepishly apologize for talking about a treatment that everyone knows does nothing! I personally do not believe that a forced intake of calcium will have any beneficial effect on osteoporosis in an individual who has been on a reasonably balanced diet.

While most vitamins and minerals are harmless if taken in recommended doses, there are certain ones that should be avoided. Many vitamin preparations contain iron, and these should be avoided in everyone but women during their menstrual years. One of the most common features of cancer of the colon is a slow loss of blood, not enough to be seen in the stool or change its color. This slow ooze will, however, result in a common early symptom of this malignancy, iron deficiency anemia. The taking of supplemental iron will delay the onset of the anemia, delay the feeling of weakness or tiredness, and ultimately delay finding the tumor and removing it. Needless to say, the iron does nothing for the malignancy. Iron supplements cannot possibly be of any benefit to anyone not suffering from iron deficiency, and definitely are to be avoided in all but premenopausal women. See the chapter on blood for more about this.

There is also a theoretical reason to avoid one of the B vitamins called folic acid. It is impossible to become deficient in this vitamin with anything approaching a normal diet. Additional quantities are necessary in individuals suffering from malnutrition, or with certain kinds of anemias where red blood cells have to be produced much faster than normal. The theoretical problem with taking folic acid revolves around a not uncommon condition called pernicious anemia. This condition results in an inability of the intestine to absorb vitamin B12 from food or tablets. The consequences of vitamin B12 deficiency are two-fold, anemia and degeneration of the spinal cord. Folic acid can, to a degree, overcome the anemia problem, but not the degeneration of the spinal cord. The result then is a delay in establishing a diagnosis, which allows more degeneration of the spinal cord than would have happened if the patient became anemic.

There certainly can be no objection by anyone to the judicious use of vitamins by the general public, especially the elderly. It will prevent any chance of borderline deficiency due to a poor diet or decreased absorptive capacity. But to place any credence in the broad claims of the vitamin or health food industry is not much different from buying a bottle of snake oil from the back of a covered wagon.

The subject of diet and its relationship to cancer has become very popular recently. There seems to be a never-ending outpouring of reports that initially implicate various kinds of foods with various kinds of cancers, and then later refute the findings. The problem is that most of these studies are based either upon statistical relationships, or upon experiments with laboratory animals that are inbred to easily develop certain kinds of cancer. Anyone who believes a *statistical* relationship to be a *causative* relationship is begging to be proved wrong. Real proof for the overwhelming majority of these claims is lacking. There are those who presuppose that some day that proof will be forthcoming. I am skeptical. I see the current situation as a lot of researchers catering to public wishful thinking.

Excess fat is one of the more common health problems we face, and certainly a lot of money is spent in attempts to trim off those pounds. If you are expecting some secret to be revealed here, you are going to be disappointed, because all I am going to do is state the simple facts.

Fat is stored food. If you eat more calories than you burn, your body will lay down fat. In order to lose fat, you have to burn more calories than you eat. Unfortunately, fat has more than twice the calories of an equal weight of sugar, and it takes a lot of excercise to burn up a pound of it. If you are trying to lose weight and not succeeding, you have to consume less calories. There is nothing more to it than that. It does no good to compare your food intake with someone else's. Everyone's metabolism is different. Someone else may remain thin on a calorie intake that would make you blow up like a balloon. But that is the way it is. There is no safe pill that will reliably curb the appetite, and no safe medication to enable you to burn fat faster. You simply have to eat less. One common reason for the constant "But I don't eat that much!" that I hear, is that people do not realize that the older you get, the slower your metabolism, and the less calories you burn. The difference over the decades is substantial. If you are eating the same diet that you ate twenty years ago, you are going to gain weight.

There is one more point about losing fat I would like to make. You have no control over what part of your body is going to be thinned by weight loss. Exercise will tone muscles, and is certainly good for you, but it will have no specific effect on the fat overlying those muscles. Gadgets that heat, massage, vibrate, or roll an area of fat do nothing.

The subject of dieting also includes the popular cholesterol and triglycerides. There is an interesting paradox in the general concern over the intake of fats. The older people get, the more worried they seem to be over their blood levels of cholesterol and triglycerides, and their fat intake. That makes little sense since it takes decades for arteries to become arteriosclerotic. The "younger" you are, the more important it is. By the time you are in your late sixties or seventies it probably makes very little difference what your various blood fat values are. There is more on this subject in Chapter 13. All I will say here is that it is a good idea for everyone to limit the intake of animal fat, and for many it is critical.

Removal of excess salt from the diet is essential in many patients. Many who think they are doing that, however, are simply kidding themselves. If you are adding *any* salt to the cooking or your food, you are not on a low-salt diet. If you are eating *any* foods processed with salt, such as cold cuts or pickles, you are not on a low-salt diet.

PART TWO

CHAPTER 11

THE BLOOD

This chapter begins the second part of the book, which deals with common diseases and conditions. As with the first part, it should be valuable as a reference now, and in the future.

The field of medicine that has to do with blood and its related organs is called hematology. I am putting it first from sheer prejudice. This specialty deals with diseases affecting the blood cells, the clotting of blood, and diseases of the bone marrow, lymph glands, and spleen. There seems to be something of a mystical aura surrounding the subject of blood, and that holds true for everyone. Of all the various specialties of medicine and surgery, patients and physicians alike seem to know and understand the least about hematology. It is really not all that complicated.

Blood consists of four main elements, the three kinds of blood cells and the plasma they are floating in. I will review, briefly, these elements and the most common problems and misunderstandings relating to them.

The three kinds of blood cells are the red blood cells, the white blood cells, and the platelets.

Red blood cells are nothing more than tiny packets containing hemoglobin. Hemoglobin, a complex chemical containing iron, has the ability to pick up and bind an enormous amount of oxygen in the lungs, and then release it in the tissues throughout the body where it is needed. In adults, red blood cells are manufactured in the marrow of the flat bones. Those are the bones exclusive of the arms and legs. A red blood cell will live approximately one hundred twenty days before it dies. "Dying" means that it is removed from the body by the spleen.

The most common problem people have with blood is anemia, and all that means is an abnormally low quantity of red blood cells. *Anemia is not a disease. It is a condition that is always caused by something, and the something is often more important than the anemia itself!* In other words, if you are told you are anemic, you should also be told why. If you're not told why, ask!

Before discussing anemia, let us understand how we measure red blood cells, and learn the normal values. The quantity of red blood cells is most accurately determined by two tests called the hematocrit (hct.) and the hemoglobin (hgb.). We will use the hematocrit numbers, which indicate what percent of whole blood is red blood cells. You can roughly translate to hemoglobin by dividing by three. The normal hematocrit for a male is between 40 percent and 52 percent and for a female 36 percent to 50 percent. This difference exists because male hormones are potent stimulators of red blood cell production. Any value below 40 percent and 36 percent respectively is defined as anemia.

Symptoms of significant anemia are most commonly tiredness, fatigue, and weakness, but the presence or absence of these symptoms is dependent upon two important factors, the severity of the anemia, and how fast it develops. A slowly developing anemia will not usually cause symptoms until the hematocrit is below 30 percent, and if "very" slowly progressive, not until much lower values. A rapid drop, however, say from 46 percent to 35 percent, can cause severe symptoms.

There are three basic mechanisms by which anemia can develop. The simplest mechanism, and by far the least common, is loss of blood. You have to be actually hemorrhaging to become anemic this way. The reason is simple. The human bone marrow, if healthy and supplied with nutrients, can manufacture more than a half a pint's worth of red blood cells every day.

The second way anemia can develop is if the red blood cells die too quickly, before their alloted one hundred twenty days. It is not difficult for the bone marrow to compensate, to increase production of red blood cells, if, for example, they only live a month. But if they only live for days, or hours, then the total quantity of red blood cells falls, and the patient becomes anemic. These kinds of anemias, and remember, so far we are only discussing a mechanism, are called hemolytic anemias.

There are many, many different kinds of hemolytic anemias. Some of them are congenital, due to a defect in the genes. People are born with them and they are passed on from one generation to the next. Others are acquired, a disease that develops. We will discuss a few examples, but first, a brief review of genes and inheritance is necessary to understand how the congenital forms are inherited.

We have two genes for every characteristic. One we get from our mother, the other from our father. If having one gene for a trait will allow that trait to develop, it is called dominant. Brown eyes are an example of this. If two identical genes are necessary for a trait to appear, it is called recessive, such as blue eyes. A blue-eyed person must have two blue genes. A brown-eyed person can have either one blue gene and one brown, or two brown genes. Can two brown-eyed people have a blue-eyed baby? Yes. If each parent has one blue gene, the odds are that one out of four of their babies will get a blue gene from each and have blue eyes. Let us look at a few common congenital hemolytic anemias, and also at how they are inherited.

Sickle cell anemia is probably the most well-known congentital hemolytic anemia. It occurs only in persons whose parents each have some black ancestors. Sickle cell anemia is caused by a very minor change in the hemoglobin molecule, and the effect is that the hemoglobin has a tendency to form crystals inside the red blood cell. Those crystals distort the cell into the shape of a sickle, hence the name, and they get stuck in blood vessels and destroyed. The blockage of blood vessels by sickled red blood cells is what causes the periodic outbreaks of pain in those patients. Sickle cell anemia is a recessive disease, meaning that two genes are necessary to cause the full-blown disease. If someone has only one abnormal gene, the condition is called sickle cell "trait."

Thalassemia major, also known as Cooley's anemia, is another congenital hemolytic anemia. This condition occurs chiefly in people of Italian ancestry. The problem here is a genetic inability to manufacture hemoglobin, the red blood cells dying even before they get out of the bone marrow. It is a very serious disease, and those afflicted with it do not usually live very long. Thalassemia major, like sickle cell anemia, is a recessive disease. If someone has only one abnormal gene, the condition is called thalassemia "minor." It can cause some anemia, but it is minimal and not a problem.

For a young couple to marry and have a baby with either of these diseases is a tragedy, and a preventable one. A simple blood test can reveal whether either or both of the prospective parents is carrying the sickle or thalassemia gene.

Congenital spherocytic anemia is another common, but less severe, congenital hemolytic anemia. It occurs mostly in people with northern European ancestry and, unlike the previous two, is genetically dominant, meaning that only one gene is necessary to have it. The disease is named because some of the red blood cells look like balls, spheres. This disease is fairly mild, often causes minimal anemia, and commonly is not discovered or diagnosed until late in life when some other illness makes the anemia more severe.

Perhaps the most common "acquired" hemolytic anemia is that caused by the development of autoantibodies. In a sense, the patient becomes allergic to his own red blood cells and destroys them. This "autoimmune hemolytic anemia" is often a complication of other diseases, or sometimes is brought on by medications, the person becoming allergic to the medication, which is attached to their red blood cells. Cortisone is most often used to treat this condition, usually with excellent results, although sometimes other measures are necessary.

The last, and most common, mechanism of anemia is the failure of the bone marrow to manufacture normal numbers of red blood cells. Here again there are many and varied causes.

First of all, the bone marrow is very sensitive to many kinds of illnesses. Prolonged infections or inflammatory diseases, poor kidney or liver function, conditions that cause an oversecretion or undersecretion of certain hormones, among others, will decrease the production of red blood cells and, over a period of time, cause a degree of anemia. These are called secondary anemias.

Pernicious anemia is a disease where the body cannot absorb vitamin B12 from the intestines because of a stomach defect. This lack of vitamin B12 can cause all three kinds of blood cells to become depleted. Treatment with injections of the vitamin brings everything back to normal.

Next to the secondary anemias, iron deficiency is the most common cause of anemia. Red blood cells are not produced if there is no iron available for them in the body. But remember, there are dozens and dozens of possible reasons to be anemic, and iron pills or shots will only help this one specific cause. Furthermore, a diagnosis of iron deficiency anemia is not even a complete diagnosis, because, aside from in infants, it is *always* caused by something else, and that something else is almost always a loss of iron from the body in the form of blood. It is next to impossible to develop iron deficiency anemia because of a poor diet. Iron is simply present in too many foods. Menstrual blood loss is certainly the most common way to lose blood from the body, and is the most common cause of iron deficiency anemia. Pregnancy is another way to lose iron because the fetus takes it from the mother's blood.

Slight degrees of anemia should be evaluated in light of a patient's age and sex. It is not uncommon for women, during the years they are menstruating, to have minimal degrees of anemia due to their monthly loss of iron. Hematocrits above 32 percent should not cause concern, but should be checked periodically. While there is nothing wrong with a trial of iron therapy in mildly anemic women during the years they are menstruating, women past that age, and all men of whatever age, must be tested further to determine the exact cause of their anemia. Any hematocrit below 40 percent in a male warrants a thorough search for the cause of the anemia. *Again, the cause of anemia is usually more important than the anemia itself.* You wouldn't accept a doctor simply telling you that you were "sick," and nothing more, so do not accept being told that you are "anemic," and nothing more.

Although there are literally hundreds of diseases that can cause anemia either directly or indirectly, ninety-nine percent of the time it is due to one of just a few common conditions. How does a doctor begin the process of sorting out which of the many diseases is causing a particular patient's anemia? He begins at the beginning, with the history, physical examination, and a routine series of blood tests. This gives him information on the great bulk of diseases that may or may not be present. The next thing he does is to look at the blood cells, the bone marrow cells, which make blood cells (and where iron is stored), and a test called a reticulocyte count that tells him how fast red blood cells are being produced. By this time, he either has the diagnosis, or has narrowed it down to just a few possibilities. It is simple!

Before leaving the red blood cell, let us have a look at the opposite of anemia, polycythemia, too many red blood cells. Patients with this condition have a hematocrit above 52 percent. I have seen a hematocrit as high as 72 percent. The blood was almost like jelly!

An abnormally high number of red blood cells can be caused by many conditions. One of the simplest is living at a very high altitude. The body compensates for the relative lack of oxygen by making more red blood cells. The most common disease that causes it, however, is called polycythemia vera, or "true" polycythemia. In this disease, the bone marrow sort of runs wild, overproducing red blood cells, and sometimes the other blood cells as well. Treatment usually consists of just removing the blood a pint at a time until the hematocrit is normal. Although periodic removal continues to be necessary, eventually the body runs out of iron, and the rate of red blood cell production falls. Untreated polycythemia can cause a whole host of problems including the formation of clots, strokes, and heart attacks. This is an easy disease to take care of, yet, a few years ago I saw a patient in the coronary care unit of a hospital where he had been admitted with a heart attack and heart failure, and a hematocrit in the mid-sixties. He knew he had polycythemia, and had been treated for it many years earlier, but then had decided to ignore it!

White blood cells exist to fight infection. They are the defenders of our body, destroying microbial invaders. A normal white blood cell count is between 5,000 and 10,000 per cubic millimeter of blood, although many black people can have normal white counts as low as 4,000, or sometimes even less. There are several different kinds of white blood cells. Some of them are involved with the immune system and the production of antibodies that bind to germs and either kill them or render them harmless. Others actually eat germs, clearing them out of the body. There is one thing white blood cells do not really do, despite a common opinion to the contrary. They do not "eat" red blood cells.

Diseases of white blood cells are concerned with their absence (leukopenia), lack of function (as in AIDS), or malignancies (the leukemias).

Diseases that cause too few white blood cells are usually those that destroy the normal bone marrow by replacing it with abnormal cells. The common end effect of any cause of too few normal white blood cells is an increased susceptibility to infection.

I am not going to get into the subject of leukemia very deeply. There are many kinds. All are manifested by the overproduction of white blood cells. In the acute leukemias, the white blood cells are markedly abnormal, have no value in fighting infection, and can cause death quickly. Recent years have shown some significant advances in the treatment of the most common acute leukemia of children. In the chronic leukemias, the white blood cells that are overproduced are near normal. Infection is much less of a problem, and in some types, the patient may live long enough to die of something else. That is especially true in the most common leukemia, called chronic lymphocytic leukemia. It is a disease mostly striking the elderly, and many patients do not even have to be treated for it for many, many years.

Platelets are very tiny blood cells that stop you from bleeding. They are, in a sense, sticky. Most people believe that it is the clotting of blood that stops the bleeding from a cut or a wound. In fact, platelets plug up the holes in the blood vessels; only after that does the blood clot.

Platelets live about ten days, and the normal platelet count ranges between approximately 170,000 and 400,000 per cubic millimeter of blood. There are conditions where the platelets become increased, but usually they are not too serious. There is a danger of developing clots or phlebitis if the platelet count rises over one million, but there are medications to both prevent clots from forming, and to lower the platelet count.

Lower than normal platelet counts can become a real problem. A count of approximately 50,000 is necessary to stop bleeding normally.

Fewer platelets than that cause abnormal bleeding. There is more on this later in this chapter.

Any disease that destroys the bone marrow will decrease the number of platelets. Indeed, patients with a destroyed bone marrow either die of infection from too few white blood cells, or from bleeding from too few platelets.

A fairly common disease that causes abnormally low platelets is called idiopathic thrombocytopenic purpura (ITP). Let me explain that name. "Idiopathic" simply means of unknown cause; "thrombocyte" is another name for a platelet (literally, clot cell); "purpura" is just another name for black-and-blue marks. ITP is another autoimmune disease, very similar to acquired hemolytic anemia, described earlier. In this case, the antibodies are against platelets instead of red blood cells. ITP often strikes children, the skin becoming covered with minute pinhead-size hemorrhages. Fortunately, in children the disease usually goes away, and is controllable with cortisone until it does. It sometimes becomes a chronic disease in adults, and is treated with cortisone, other drugs, and sometimes by removing the spleen.

Platelets very likely play another role in disease. They are thought to possibly begin the process of having a stroke or heart attack by sticking to damaged areas of blood vessels. A clot then forms around them and blocks the blood vessel. That is the reason many patients take aspirin or dipyrimadole. Those two medications make platelets less sticky.

Plasma is the fluid part of blood. It consists of two basic components: serum, and the factors that make blood clot. In other words, if you allow blood, or plasma, to form a clot, the liquid that is left over is serum. Serum consists of a multitude of proteins, lipids, and a whole host of chemicals, dissolved in water.

Clotting is a very complex process that involves several different specific proteins and lipids, as well as other chemicals. The chain of chemical reactions that leads to a clot can be started by either plasma touching a foreign surface, or by the introduction of certain tissue substances. As mentioned in Chapter 8, many patients take warfarin to inhibit the clotting of blood. It sort of slows the process down.

Hemophilia and related conditions are congenital disorders of clotting. Patients affected are missing one of the clotting proteins that I mentioned above. The hemophiliac will stop bleeding from a cut in a normal amount of time since his platelets are normal. The problem is that the platelet "plug" does not last long, and without a clot forming behind it, bleeding soon begins again. Hemophilia, and its almost identical sister condition, Christmas disease, are inherited on the X sex chromosone. Men have only one X, so if it carries the gene, they have the disease. Women have two X chromosomes, and even when they have the gene on one, the other is almost invariably normal. These women do not have the disease but they are carriers. There are concentrates of clotting factors available for treating just about all the congenital clotting deficiencies.

The kind of abnormal bleeding one sees in patients with hemophilia, or any other clotting disorder, is quite different from that seen in patients with very low platelet counts. Hemophiliacs classically bleed internally, into joints or body cavities. Patients with low platelets usually bleed under the skin, or from the nose and gums.

Let us continue on with this subject of bleeding. The most common cause of a tendency to bleed abnormally is aspirin. As I stated above, aspirin makes platelets less sticky, and it prolongs bleeding. The effect can last as long as ten days or more. While many patients take aspirin for this very reason, it is a good idea to stay away from it for a couple of weeks if you are going to have surgery.

I often see patients referred to me because they are concerned about their black-and-blue marks, and they are almost always women. The fact is that women simply bruise more easily than men. Female blood vessels are more fragile than those in the male and break more easily. Do not be concerned if you have occasional black-and-blue marks, even several at one time. Staying away from aspirin will help. See a doctor if there are more than a dozen or so on your body at any one time, and especially if there is an associated bleeding from your nose or gums.

Elderly patients, again particularly women, are even more prone to bleeding under the skin. Blood vessels and the tissues that support them become more fragile as you get older. Sometimes elderly women develop large red blotches on their arms and legs. It may be an unsightly problem, but it is not usually a serious one. If you are concerned, a few simple blood tests can determine that your platelets and clotting chemicals are normal.

Finally, what do you do if you are bleeding from a cut, or your nose? The answer is simple. Press on it, and keep the pressure on. Your finger can exert more pressure than the blood in the vessel, and collapse it. When it is the nose, a substantial cylinder of tissue paper shoved into the nostril will give you something to press against.

Lymph glands are where a certain kind of white blood cell called lymphocytes are made. Do not confuse lymph glands with glands that produce hormones. Lymph glands are scattered all over the body, and also serve as barriers against the spread of infection. When you get a sore throat and the glands in your neck are enlarged and painful, those are lymph glands. Second to infections, most diseases of lymph glands are malignancies. These include Hodgkins disease and lymphomas or lymphosarcomas.

The spleen is an organ about the size of a fist located in the left upper part of the abdomen, tucked up under the ribs. It serves as a blood-cell producing organ in fetuses and perhaps young babies, and as an important part of the immune system in children. In adults, the spleen acts mainly as a blood filter, removing old blood cells from the circulation. The most common problem with spleens involves their enlargement. Infections such as infectious mononucleosis, liver diseases (especially cirrhosis), malignancies of lymph glands, and certain bone marrow diseases, all cause the spleen to become enlarged. The latter conditions can make it grow to the size of a football! An enlarged spleen, in and of itself, is usually not a major problem unless a condition called hypersplenism develops. As you might guess, hypersplenism means an overfunctioning of the spleen. Instead of removing only old or damaged blood cells from the blood, young and normal cells are removed also. Any one, or two, or all three types of blood cells may be affected. Most of the time the counts do not become low enough to be dangerous, but when they do, the spleen must be removed.

CHAPTER 12

ARTHRITIS, AND ACHES
AND PAINS

A*rthritis* seems to have become an almost universal term among patients for all manner of aches and pains. That is unfortunate because there also appears to be an accompanying opinion that little can be done for it, almost a feeling of helplessness. True arthritis is one cause, but not the most common cause, of aches and pains in the patients I have seen over the years.

Arthritis is the inflammation of a joint. In case you are not sure what joints are, they are the movable connections between two bones. They include the ankles, knees, hips, knuckles, elbows, and shoulders. Arthritis is inflammation *inside* those joints, and is usually characterized by pain, swelling, heat, perhaps even some redness. Yet, it is not uncommon for patients to state with authority that the pain in their leg or thigh is due to arthritis, even when their hips, knees, and ankles are obviously normal. Pains in the extremities can be a result of arthritis but not in the way most people suppose. More on that a little later.

I see three major reasons for all this confusion. One is that the most common form of arthritis, osteoarthritis, is indeed very common, almost universal, in the elderly. The second is that X-rays of the spine, in almost everybody past the point of being young, will reveal bone changes that radiologists call osteoarthritic. These bone changes, however, are most often *not* the cause of the pain. It is only natural, I guess, that such frequent use of the word results in its becoming used even when erroneous. The third reason is that aches and pains resulting from many different causes are often treated with anti-inflammatory medication, otherwise known as arthritis pills.

We will discuss true arthritis, then those parts of the body that give us the most discomfort, and the real reasons for it.

As previously stated, osteoarthritis is by far the most common form of arthritis. These degenerative changes in the joints affect us all as we grow older. The more common joints affected are the knees, fingers (especially the last joint, near the nail, which gets knobby as the arthritis progresses), hips, and of course the spine. But remember, with one kind of exception, the pain from osteoarthritis is *in* the joint, not just near it!

The exception I mentioned is when osteoarthritis of the spine causes such severe thickening of the spinal bones that they compress the nerves coming out of the spinal cord. The pain that is caused by irritation of these nerves is called a radicular pain. Many patients are confused by this concept. They cannot understand how a back problem, for example, can cause pain in a leg. The sensations of pain are transmitted through nerves. If the root of the nerve is irritated, you feel the pain in the part of the body that root goes to. If you are still confused, look at it this way. If you touch a battery to a wire, it is the light bulb at the end of the wire that lights up, not the wire itself. You can get a radicular pain originating in the lower spine, which causes pain that shoots into your buttock and leg, or in the upper spine in your neck, which causes pain that shoots into your shoulder or arm. This thickening osteoarthritis of the spine is not the only cause of that type of pain. Slipped or herniated discs are another major cause. There is more on that condition later.

The treatment for osteoarthritis is not all we would like it to be. Aspirin and other anti-inflammatory medications do help most people at least to some degree. Getting rid of excess pounds of fat can lessen the wear and tear on an involved knee or hip, and that can be quite important. When such joints are severely affected, they can be surgically replaced. Spinal surgery to relieve the pressure on the nerves is indicated for patients with severe radicular pain from thickened spinal bones.

Rheumatoid arthritis is a very painful disease that, if severe, results in the destruction of the joints it affects. It is also treated with anti-inflammatory drugs, but also with cortisone, gold, even potent immunosuppressive drugs. Patients suffering from a severe case of rheumatoid arthritis should probably be under the care of a specialist, a rheumatologist.

There is a host of other causes of arthritis. These include infections (including gonorrhea), psoriasis, ileitis (an inflammatory disease of the small intestine), and an autoimmune disease called systemic lupus erythematosis, among others. It is beyond the scope of this book to discuss them all. I will, however, discuss one other, gout. It is not extremely common, but those who have it are invariably confused about the way it is treated.

The inflammation in gout is caused by the deposition of uric acid crystals into the joint, and it is horrendously painful. Uric acid is a normal chemical in the blood. It is a waste product that is excreted in the urine. Although most patients with gout will have abnormally high amounts of uric acid in the blood, not all do. Likewise, having high amounts of uric acid does not mean you are going to get gout, only that you are more predisposed to it.

The classic place to get gout is at the base of a big toe. That is called podagra, an acute severe arthritis. Other joints may also be affected. It is treated with the more potent anti-inflammatory drugs, which are very effective in this disorder. If you have only had gout once, or get an attack very infrequently, there is no other treatment indicated. If, however, you get attacks of gout frequently there is another way to treat the condition, to *prevent* the attacks. That medication is called, generically, allopurinol.

Allopurinol has no affect on a joint that is inflamed by gout, but it does decrease the formation of uric acid in the body, and lowers the total amount in the blood, and in the body, *over a period of time*. Once you have taken allopurinol for several months, you will probably never have an attack of gout again, if you keep taking it. During those first several months, however, your chances of having another attack may be increased! That problem is usually overcome by taking yet another medication during those months, colchicine. Colchicine is also effective in treating the acute arthritis of gout, but it can cause severe diarrhea. Much smaller doses that do *not* usually cause diarrhea, however, can prevent acute attacks of gout until the allopurinol has had its full effect. I know it is confusing, but there is a little more to come. Treatment with allopurinol may be indicated for reasons other than having frequent attacks of gout. These include having an *excessively* high level of uric acid in the blood, being predisposed to forming uric acid stones in the kidneys (not calcium stones), and having visible deposits, called tophaceous gout, in the bones, joints, or ears. Patients receiving chemotherapy for certain kinds of malignancies, especially leukemia, are put on allopurinol because of their tendency to develop very high levels of uric acid and gout.

One note of caution about allopurinol. Patients often become allergic to it, as many as one out of twenty.

There is another, uncommon, disease that fits into the category of the arthritides even though it is not a true arthritis. It is called polymyalgia rheumatica (poly-, many; my-, muscle; -algia, pain; rheumatica, rheumatism, which is a nonspecific term meaning bodily aches and pains). I see about one case every two years. Polymyalgia rheumatica causes pain, sometimes very severe, in the proximal muscles, meaning the thighs, buttocks, and upper arms. It can also cause pain, but not inflammation, in some joints, usually the fingers. Anti-inflammatory medication seems to have no effect on this condition at all, but it responds very well to cortisone, usually only requiring a short period of treatment.

Many patients come to my office complaining of a vague earache that turns out to be pain due to arthritis of the joint between the mandible (the jaw bone) and the temporal bone of the skull. This temporomandibular joint is located just in front of the ear, and becomes inflamed and painful usually from either dental problems or nocturnal grinding of the teeth. Anti-inflammatory medication helps. Sometimes using a bite plate, fitted by a dentist, at night is necessary.

Let us turn our attention to the parts of the body that seem to give us humans the most pain and discomfort, and see what else causes pain other than arthritis.

In my experience the most common cause of neck pain, by far, is simply anxiety, nervous tension. In a great many of us, nervous tension results in the chronic *and involuntary* contraction of various muscles. If you want to know how painful that can be, just hold your arm straight out away from you for five minutes. See if you can do it! This kind of tension is a common cause of headaches in the forehead and temples when the scalp muscles are affected. If the muscles in the back of the neck are chronically contracted, it can cause pain anywhere from the base of the skull and neck to the backs of the shoulders and the back itself. Do not forget, when X-rays of the neck are taken, they will likely show osteoarthritic changes, but that does not prove that the arthritic changes are causing the pain! Sometimes some firm pressing or squeezing with your fingers may reveal that the area is far more tender than muscles elsewhere in your body. Other than getting rid of your anxiety by changing your life, the best treatment I have found is a combination of an over-the-counter painkiller taken with a small dose of a tranquilizer. Tranquilizers, incidentally, are the best muscle relaxants.

While we are on the upper back, I should mention a condition called subscapular bursitis. A scapula is a shoulder blade. A bursa is a small fluid-filled sack that tendons move over. There is one under each scapula that can cause a sharp pain when inflamed. If you have this condition, you will probably find that you cannot really point exactly to the pain and that nothing in the area is tender. That is because it is under the bone. Put your hand of the side that is affected across your chest onto the opposite shoulder. That moves the scapula out of the way. Now, if somebody pokes in the area of the pain, you will probably find a spot of tenderness. If the pain is not severe, bear with it. It might go away by itself. If it is severe or persistent, I treat it with an injection of a small amount of cortisone into the bursa.

Shoulder pain is a common complaint, yet in eighteen years in practice I have seen very few cases of true arthritis of the shoulder. The most common cause of shoulder pain, and by that I mean pain in the shoulder that is aggravated by moving the arm or lying on it, is called calcific tendinitis, or capsulitis, or bursitis. The pain is caused by inflammation around tiny deposits of calcium in the muscles or tendons.

Most of the time these deposits are too small to be seen on an X-ray. We all have them, I am sure. I think they are caused by lack of use of the muscles. How often, for example, do we use the muscles that bring our elbows above the height of our shoulders? It is not uncommon for pain from this condition to appear after trauma, such as an automobile accident, or after using the arms vigorously, such as when shoveling snow. The calcium deposits have been there all along, but now the unusual activity incites the inflammation. Capsulitis can be treated with anti-inflammatory medication, cortisone shots, and exercise, but there is another form of treatment I was recently introduced to that is extremely effective. More on that later.

Chest pain coming from the heart will be discussed in that chapter, but there are three other common causes of chest pain. Two of those three are discussed in the chapter on the gastrointestinal system, namely a hiatus hernia and gas. The third belongs here.

Costochondritis is among the most common causes of chest pain, and definitely is the most common for chest pain in young women. The pain, which can be very severe, comes from inflammation of joints where the ribs join the sternum (chest bone). The ribs and sternum are separated by cartilage, hence the name (costo- refers to ribs, and chond- refers to cartilage). The pain is usually between the nipple line and the center of the chest, and for some reason is far more common on the left.

Costochondritis can be caused by chronic contraction of the muscles between the ribs from anxiety, or by excessive breathing and sighing (hyperventilating), which is also caused by anxiety. The hyperventilation syndrome is discussed in the chapter on psychosomatic disorders. You can test yourself for this condition by pressing firmly where it hurts. See if the area is more tender than other spots on the chest. If you have chest pain, however, the wisest course is to check it out with your doctor. Costochondritis is usually treated with anti-inflammatory medication, but the treatment I alluded to earlier, and will discuss later, is extremely effective.

Low-back problems are the price we pay for walking on two feet. The human species has not yet fully evolved the anatomy to do that to perfection. There are a myriad of causes for low-back pain, but the most common are due to strains of muscles and ligaments. I have found the most common causes are lifting objects improperly, slouching in a chair, and especially reading or watching television in bed while propped up on pillows. Analgesics and muscle relaxants are usually prescribed, although elimination of bad posture habits usually results in a lessening and disappearance of the pain, after a while. More on treatment of these conditions later.

Sciatica, or sciatic neuritis, is the inflammation of a specific nerve. It causes a pain that originates in the buttock and radiates down the back of the leg. It is a difficult condition to treat. Sometimes anti-inflammatory medication helps, sometimes not. Fortunately, it usually goes away by itself, but perhaps not until quite some time has passed.

There is another cause for buttock pain that has become more frequent during recent years, and that is credit cards. More specifically, credit cards in a wallet that you carry in a hip pocket. Sitting on that relatively hard object can result in a great deal of pain, most patients not making the connection until it is pointed out to them.

Elderly patients, particularly women, and often those not so elderly, frequently develop severe pain along the upper margin of the buttocks, sometimes in the buttocks themselves. It can be quite severe, even incapacitating. I am not certain as to the cause, only that it is a muscular pain, and that it responds to the type of treatment I will now discuss.

Over a year ago, I tried out a machine that emits a pulsating electromagnetic field. I am not one for gadgets, but when the salesman showed me a picture of it, I remembered seeing it being used by some Scandinavian athletes on television during the summer Olympics. Being completely unable to throw at the time because of shoulder problems, I took the machine on a one-month-trial basis and used it on my shoulder. To my utter surprise and delight, every treatment melted more and more pain away. I have not used it now for over a year, but I throw with no discomfort at all, although I still cannot get a fastball past my son.

I have used that machine now on hundreds of patients; and for capsulitis of the shoulder, costochondritis, the usual causes of low-back pain, the buttock pain I mentioned just above, and pain from injuries, it is extremely effective. I have even used it on two patients suffering from chest-wall pain following coronary artery bypass surgery, and the pain disappeared in both.

I have tried the machine on two other painful conditions that are essentially untreatable. I am going to mention them with great hesitancy because the numbers have been very few, and because I find the results hard to believe myself. Many patients who have had shingles (see the chapter on infections) suffer from pain long after the shingles has healed. I used the machine on three patients who were suffering from this pain for up to three years, and the pain either disappeared or markedly lessened in all three. I also tried the machine in two patients who seemed to be suffering from diabetic neuropathy (a painful nerve complication of diabetes), and both reported a marked reduction in their pain.

The machine is not a panacea. I have not seen it help true arthritis, nor sciatic neuritis, but to say that I strongly recommend it for the other conditions mentioned above is putting it mildly. My wife understands that when the day comes that I retire, that machine is staying with us!

The last topic for this chapter is herniated discs. The bones of the spinal column are separated from each other by discs. Each has a fibrous shell and a gelatinlike core. They are sort of like shock absorbers, and allow the spinal column to flex and bend. Sometimes, the fibrous shell breaks down and the gelatin protrudes, or herniates. The problems arise when this protruding gelatin presses on nerves or nerve roots coming out of the spinal cord and causes a radicular pain. The lumbar (lower) spine is more commonly affected, but some times a disc in the cervical (neck) spine can herniate.

Discs cannot be seen on an X-ray. If an X-ray reveals that the space between two spinal bones is markedly narrowed, the presence of a herniated disc can be inferred. In order to really see a herniated disc, either a myelogram (an X-ray of the spine after a contrast material has been injected into the spinal fluid) or a CAT scan must be done.

There are various treatments for herniated discs including anti-inflammatory medications, rest, injections, and traction. I am not expert enough to discuss them since I usually send my patients with these problems to an orthopedist or a neurosurgeon. The ultimate treatment for a herniated disc is surgery.

*   *   *

Remember, if you are going to the doctor because of an ache or a pain, know for certain exactly where it hurts, and do not be careless with names for parts of the body. Do not mislead him.

CHAPTER 13

ARTERIES AND VEINS

Having a problem with their "circulation" is a common concern of many patients. Some are thoroughly convinced they have such a condition when there is nothing wrong with their blood vessels at all. Although many people use the term, few really have much of an understanding of what it means or the diseases involved. If you want to understand problems with the circulation, you first have to understand the circulation, and the very basic difference between arteries and veins.

Arteries are thick-walled vessels that carry blood away from the heart to the tissues of the body. The blood in arteries is rich in oxygen and nutrients, and is under high pressure. When we use the term blood pressure, we really mean arterial blood pressure. Picture arteries as the water pipes in your home. Veins are thin-walled vessels. They carry the blood back to the heart. This blood is poor in oxygen and nutrients, and is under very low pressure. Picture veins sort of like the drainpipe of your sink. The network of microscopic blood vessels that connect the smallest arteries (the arterioles) and the smallest veins (the venules) are called capillaries.

The difference in the pressure in arteries and veins, and the fact that it is the arteries that supply oxygen and food to all the tissues of the body, makes the diseases of these two kinds of blood vessels quite different. We will discuss arteries first.

The most common disease of arteries is arteriosclerosis, hardening of the arteries. The problem is not so much that the arteries get hard, but rather that they get much narrower because of the deposition of fat in the walls. It is obvious that less water will flow through a half-inch-diameter pipe than a one-inch. When the internal size of an artery gets too small, the tissues it supplies with blood begin to suffer from a lack of oxygen. This is called ischemia. The parts of the body that are most commonly affected by ischemia are the legs, heart, and brain. The heart is discussed in the chapter dealing with that organ, and the brain in the miscellaneous chapter. We will confine our discussion here to the legs.

The earliest symptoms of an inadequate blood supply to the legs usually occur when the most oxygen is needed, in other words, when the muscles are used. The person will experience a tightening or cramping pain when walking, usually in the calf, called claudication. If the condition progresses, the pain comes with less and less exertion until the point is reached where there may be continual pain. Past that point, the tissues begin to die and gangrene sets in.

There are different forms of hardening of the arteries. Sometimes only a very short segment of a large artery is severely affected. Other times the entire large artery is severely diseased. In diabetics the condition commonly affects the smallest arteries most severely. This is important when it comes to treating the condition.

The first aspect of treating arteriosclerosis is prevention, to whatever degree that is possible. Understand that arteriosclerosis is part of the aging process, and that it happens to everyone, the only difference being how fast the process progresses, at what age problems occur. There are many factors that are believed to contribute to arteriosclerosis. Blood levels of cholesterol and triglycerides have received much attention in recent years. Let us look at that for a moment.

Some of us live to a ripe old age and die of a disease unrelated to hardening of the arteries. Others of us drop dead at a young age because fats clog the arteries in our hearts. Is this difference diet related? Can it be shown that *all* the former have lived on vegetables, and *all* the latter on beef and butter? Absolutely not! But the relationship between animal fat intake and the development of severe hardening of the arteries *can* be shown on a *statistical* basis, in other words, only when enough of us are studied to show what fats do, *on the average*, to the human species.

Since we are dealing with averages, it follows that in some of us diet has very little to do with the health of our arteries, in others of us it is a factor of some significance, and in still others, it is crucial, a matter of life or death.

Why is it that fats are detrimental to humans? And why does the progression of arteriosclerosis vary so greatly from one person to another? Let us take a look at other animals. If you feed a high-fat diet to a dog, nothing much happens. If you feed it to a rabbit, you can almost watch its arteries clog up. The difference between the two is simply in their inherited metabolism, the enzymes in their body and blood that affect their ability to effectively handle fat without having it become deposited in their arteries. Man is decended from animals that were probably chiefly herbivorous. Man alone of the great apes became a hunter, and began to consume large quantities of animal fat. Those least able to tolerate it died off quickly. Those able to do so better lived longer and reproduced more. At the present point in our evolution, we have acquired the ability to metabolize fats better than a rabbit, but not as well as a dog. It is not hard to see that in this state of flux, there should be significant individual variation in our ability to tolerate animal fat.

A high-fat diet is certainly no good for anyone, but if there is no history of early problems with hardening of the arteries in your family, I doubt that a "reasonable" fat intake is going to do you any harm. If, however, arteriosclerotic-type diseases are prevalent in your blood relatives, I would suggest staying away from animal fats completely. And remember, contrary to what seems to be the popular impression, the younger you are, the more important it is.

There are other factors that contribute to arteriosclerosis besides your genes. Diabetes, high blood pressure, and smoking play a role. You cannot do anything about your genes, but you can make certain you have normal blood pressure, blood sugar, blood fats, and do not smoke.

Treatment of insufficient blood supply to the legs has two aspects, medical and surgical. Medical treatment consists of medication, which will increase the blood supply to a degree, and exercise. Exercise has the effect of promoting the development of alternate circulation in the affected area. If medical treatment is insufficient, then the situation calls for vascular surgery, if possible. As mentioned earlier, often it is only a short segment of a large artery that is severely blocked. If that is the case, the blocked portion can be bypassed by a vascular surgeon. The only way to determine if such surgery is possible is to have an arteriogram. Most often such bypass procedures are simple, quick, and are profoundly successful. Unfortunately, many times no corrective surgery is possible. That is often the case in diabetics, where the hardening and narrowing process affects chiefly the small arteries. If the disease becomes severe, and tissues begin to die, amputation is the only recourse.

On occasion an artery will become blocked by a different process, an embolus. An embolus is simply a clot that has formed in one place and moves through the blood vessels to another. In the case of an arterial embolus, the clot usually forms in the heart, and travels through ever smaller arteries until it gets lodged somewhere. This can completely cut off the blood supply. The treatment is an emergency embolectomy, removal of the embolus, and anticoagulation to slow down the clotting process of the blood.

Fat deposits in the wall of an artery deteriorate and weaken it, and sometimes that results in a dilation of the artery. This is called an aneurysm. The danger of an aneurysm is that since the blood in arteries is under high pressure, the artery can rupture if the wall is weakened sufficiently.

The aorta, the major artery leaving the heart, is most commonly subject to the formation of an aneurysm, especially in the abdomen. Aneurysms take a long time to form, and during the early stages there are no symptoms. Pain, either in the abdomen or in the back, is commonly a warning sign that an aneurysm is soon to rupture. That unhappy event can come about quite quickly. I will never forget the man who came to my office about fifteen years ago complaining of a very mild abdominal pain. His aortic aneurysm was easily palpable and tender. I insisted that he see a vascular surgeon immediately. As I was saying this to him, the man's wife kept looking at me as if I were crazy, so I told them how Albert Einstein had died within minutes from a ruptured aortic aneurysm. The man did go to see the surgeon, and arrangements were made for his admission to the hospital. Before he was admitted, however, his pain markedly worsened. He called the surgeon, got to the hospital, and they opened him up just as his aneurysm was rupturing. A ten or fifteen minute delay would have meant his death, but he is still with us.

One more word about arteries. Many people experience painful leg or foot cramps at night. Sometimes they wake up in severe pain, their toes curling one way or the other. This problem is almost never caused by problems with circulation. See Chapter 23.

Diseases of veins are, for the most part, confined to the lower legs. Since the function of these vessels does not involve carrying oxygen to the muscles, the symptoms are totally different. Also, a distinction must also be made between the superficial veins of the legs, those right under the skin, and the deep big veins, the ones you cannot see.

The most common problem involving veins is the development of varicosities. A varicose vein is simply one that has dilated, been stretched into a larger size. Remember, veins have much thinner and weaker walls than arteries. The veins in your legs have valves in them, like flaps, which support segments of the long column of blood in your veins when you are standing. Once these veins begin to dilate, however, the valves no longer work, and all the weight of the blood, from the height of your heart, is pressing on the veins in your lower legs, making them dilate even more. The most common reason to begin developing dilated veins or varicosities is pregnancy. The large heavy uterus presses on the big veins in the abdomen and partially blocks the flow of blood. That is why women suffer from this condition more than men, although men can get it also. When the superficial veins in your leg develop varicosities, you see them as bluish bulges under the skin.

The best way to control the development of varicose veins is to wear support stockings, and to lie down a few times a day for a half hour or so and raise your feet above head level to allow the blood to drain out.

Phlebitis is another common problem affecting the veins in the legs. The word literally means inflammation of a vein. It is commonly called thrombophlebitis because there is usually a clot in the vein. Clots form in the slowly moving blood inside veins much more readily than in the rapidly moving blood inside arteries. It is this disease that makes the distinction between superficial and deep veins so important.

Superficial thrombophlebitis results in a painful area of the leg that may be red and is tender to the touch. You may even feel something hard that is the clot in the vein. The condition usually arises in varicosities, and is due to damage to the internal lining of the veins. Treatment consists of keeping the legs elevated and a lot of wet heat. Sometimes, anti-inflammatory medication is prescribed to lessen the pain. In this condition, there is no danger of the clots embolizing, moving to some other part of the body. There is however, the potential to develop skin ulcers and cellulitis (infection of the skin). There is more on this subject in the chapters dealing with edema and infection.

Deep vein thrombophlebitis is a different story. This condition causes pain in the calf that is worsened by standing, and relieved, at least to a degree, by reclining. Unlike arterial disease, which causes more pain when walking, and usually less or no pain when standing still or sitting, deep vein phlebitis pain is usually worst when standing still or sitting. These big veins do have clots in them that can break free and travel through the veins to the lungs. This is called a pulmonary embolus, and is discussed in the chapter on the lungs. Patients who have a lot of pain from deep vein thrombophlebitis are the fortunate ones. The inflammation that causes the pain also makes the clot adhere more firmly to the vein and makes an embolus less likely. Little or no pain means there is little or no inflammation, and that makes it very possible that a clot will break free. This is an insidious and sometimes fatal disease. Beware of the slight discomfort in your calf that goes away when you lie down! Be sure to see your doctor about it.

The treatment of deep vein thrombophlebitis consists of bed rest, leg elevation, anticoagulation, and heat. It is a slow process, and complete healing takes many weeks.

CHAPTER 14

THE HEART

The heart is nothing but a convoluted muscle, not much different from the muscles in your arms or legs. This muscle, however, functions as a pump. It normally contracts sixty to a hundred times per minute, forcing blood to flow throughout the body. The force of the expulsion of blood from the heart is felt in the arteries as a pulse. Like other pumps, the heart has valves, basically check valves, to allow the blood to flow in only one direction. And like other muscles, the heart has its own arteries within its muscle to supply blood to nourish it.

I am sure most of you know that the heart has four chambers, but we will review that briefly. The smaller chambers are called the atria. They receive venous blood returning to the heart. The larger and more powerful chambers are the ventricles. They receive blood from the atria and propel it out of the heart. Let's follow blood coming from your arm veins through its journey through the heart and back out again. Your blood enters the right atrium, then passes through the tricuspid valve into the right ventricle. From there it is propelled through the pulmonary valve into the lungs. The venous blood from the lungs enters the left atrium, passes through the bicuspid or mitral valve into the left ventricle, which pumps it past the aortic valve into the aorta, and from there throughout the rest of your body, including your arm.

When I stated that the normal heart rate is between sixty and one hundred beats per minute, I was referring to a normal "resting" heart rate. When our bodies need more blood, such as when exercising, the heart rate increases to pump more blood. Exercise, however, is not the only thing that increases the heart rate. Fear and anxiety do also.

In order for a heart to pump effectively, it has to contract in a coordinated manner that will most efficiently eject the blood. This is accomplished by what is almost an independent nervous or wiring system within the heart called the conducting system. The stimulus (think of it as being electrical) that makes a heart contract begins in a spot in the right atrium called the SA node. All parts of the heart can stimulate it to beat, but the SA node does it the fastest (sixty to one hundred times per minute), so it is the normal pacesetter, the controlling pacemaker. This stimulus travels throughout the atria, but can enter the ventricles in only one spot, the AV node. The stimulus is delayed at the AV node for a fraction of a second, then it is conducted through special fibers throughout the ventricles, causing them to contract.

Diseases of the heart affect either the valves, the arteries supplying its muscle with blood, the electrical conducting system, the muscle itself, or the sack the heart sits in (the pericardium). Let us have a look at the more common ones.

Most conditions that seriously affect the valves are the consequences of other diseases, such as rheumatic fever, arteriosclerosis, and heart attacks, or from congenital malformation. A damaged valve will either not be able to open fully (stenosis) or close fully (insufficient). One consequence of having a heart valve problem is that you will have a "murmur," which brings us to an area of confusion. What exactly is a murmur?

A murmur is nothing more than a noise made by the blood flowing through the heart. It is much the same as when you hear water flowing through the pipes in your home. There is something more about that noise made in the heart that is important to keep in mind. It must be "loud enough" to be heard by a human ear with the aid of a stethoscope. Everyone's heart makes noise, but our ears are not sensitive enough to hear this "normal" noise, most of the time. If the human ear were more sensitive, everyone would have a murmur. Now remember, I said we cannot hear normal heart noises "most of the time."

Murmurs are only of concern for one of two reasons. The first is if the murmur is being caused by a *significant* defect in a valve that causes a *significant* problem with the heart's pumping action. If a valve does not fully open, or does not fully close, there may be a serious change in the pressure inside any of the four heart chambers. If that is the case, the valve can be fixed or replaced when necessary.

The second cause for concern is that if a valve is damaged, it can become infected, even if the damage itself is minor. An infected heart valve (endocarditis) is very serious business. That is why when it is recommended that you take an antibiotic even for routine dental procedures, do it! Germs commonly enter the blood from dental work, and under normal circumstances are quickly killed off. If one happens to lodge on a damaged heart valve, however, it can find a home, begin to reproduce, and cause an infection.

That brings us to the subject of murmurs that can be heard in normal hearts. These are sometimes called hemic, or flow, murmurs. All it means is that for some reason, perhaps fever, perhaps an underlying anxiety that makes the heart contract more forcefully, or perhaps simply because of a thin chest wall, a normal heart noise becomes loud enough to be heard. The most serious problem with this kind of murmur is that some people develop a fixation. They become chronically frightened that there is something wrong with their heart despite repeated reassurances.

The most common diseases of the heart involve the arteries that supply its muscles with blood, the coronary arteries. There is a wide variation in the severity of these conditions, but they are all lumped together under the broad category of coronary heart disease or arteriosclerotic heart disease (ASHD). The basic problem is one of deposition of fats in the walls of the coronary arteries. These plaques, as they are called, narrow the vessel and obstruct the flow of blood to a varying degree. This process can be complicated by hemorrhages into these fatty deposits, which suddenly completely block the coronary artery. Various secondary names are added to ASHD depending upon the symptoms and what is happening to the heart. The most common of these are angina pectoris (or simply angina), coronary insufficiency, and acute myocardial infarction (a heart attack).

The more active the body, the more blood the heart has to pump. The more blood it has to pump, the greater the heart's own need for the blood's nutrients and oxygen. Activity of the body usually means physical exercise, but it includes even the work of digesting and absorbing food, and, again, being tense, anxious, or afraid. It is not surprising, therefore, that the usual earliest symptom of ASHD is what is called angina of effort, the common angina, heart symptoms, pain, occurring only under circumstances where the heart is working hard. In this situation the heart muscles receive enough blood when in a quiet state, but not enough when the heart has to work harder.

The most common symptom of angina is a squeezing or pressing pain in the chest, which may or may not radiate up to the neck, jaw, teeth, left shoulder, left arm, or back. Some patients may not experience the feeling in the chest at all, only in one or more of the other areas, or even the upper abdomen. Occasional patients may not experience any sensation of pain at all with angina; they may only develop a feeling of breathlessness. It is a characteristic of this common type of angina that the symptoms are brought on by exertion and relieved by resting, and often come more readily after eating.

Remember, despite what so many apprehensive people seem to think, angina is most definitely not the commonest cause of chest pain! Costochondritis (Chapter 12) and gas pain (Chapter 18) are far more common.

If and when the obstruction to the flow of blood in a coronary artery (or arteries) worsens, the symptoms become more severe. Pain and breathlessness may come with very little exertion, then with no exertion at all. This is often called coronary insufficiency. There is another mechanism to be mentioned here. Sometimes the obstruction to the flow of blood is not entirely due to deposition of fat in the arterial wall. Sometimes there is an associated spasm or contraction of the artery, which decreases its size for a while, causes symptoms, and then relaxes. This is called vasospasm.

The final consequence of this disease process is a heart attack, known, as just mentioned, as a myocardial infarction, and also as the less used term, coronary thrombosis. An infarction is the death of tissue due to deprivation of blood, and that is what happens to an area of heart muscle. The size and consequence of the infarction are dependent upon several factors. These include the size of the artery involved, the suddenness of the deprivation of blood, and the presence of what is called collateral circulation. Collateral circulation occurs when small blood vessels from another coronary artery grow into the area of heart muscle that is partially deprived of blood, thereby supplying it with more of the blood it needs. Exercise promotes the development of a collateral circulation. That is why exercise is so important.

As mentioned earlier, a blockage of a coronary artery severe enough to cause the death of the heart muscle it supplies, an infarction, can occur either by a slow gradual buildup of fat in the arterial wall, or by a sudden hemorrhage into an otherwise small fatty deposit. It is this latter event that seems to most commonly cause sudden death in younger people who seemed to have no previous heart disease. Patients who experience years of angina before they have a heart attack usually have developed a collateral circulation. This collateral circulation limits the size of the infarcted area and may prevent death from the heart attack.

Much has been said about the dangers of shoveling snow, about how many men drop dead from heart attacks while engaged in that activity. It is true, and here is why. If someone has developed a significant degree of blockage of a coronary artery, but has been leading a relatively quiet and inactive life, he may not have any symptoms. If that person were to suddenly walk briskly on a warm day, he might then experience some transient symptoms, angina. But if that person suddenly begins doing very heavy work in very cold weather, he may quickly pass the point of having only angina. He may put such a severe and unaccustomed demand on his heart that he rapidly progresses to the point of infarcting his heart muscle. The key to exercise, therefore, is to get into it very gradually. Never do anything in a sudden spurt that you are not accustomed to doing.

Most patients having a heart attack will experience severe pain in the areas mentioned above for angina. However, it is not at all uncommon for people, especially diabetics, to experience minimal or no symptoms at all of a heart attack. Many times I have had to inform patients that they had a heart attack sometime in the past. Often they do not believe it, other times they recall a transient feeling of chest discomfort or weakness months or years earlier. This is a reason that periodic electrocardiograms are important, and why any and all *new* chest symptoms, no matter the severity, should be checked out by a physician immediately.

How does a doctor know if your chest pain is angina or not? The diagnosis of angina is usually a clinical diagnosis, meaning that the specific details of your chest pain are indicative of the condition. The diagnosis can usually be confirmed by a simple trial of therapy, giving you angina medication to see if the symptoms go away. A simple electrocardiogram is often *not* helpful in making a diagnosis of angina. While there may be changes in the EKG if it is taken during the time you have your symptoms, it is often normal when you have no symptoms. That brings us to the subject of stress testing.

A stress test is basically taking your EKG while you are exercising, so the abnormalities will show up. There are also heart scans that can be done to reveal ASHD. Remember, however, none of these tests is foolproof. On occasion, each can be falsely normal or abnormal. The most reliable test for ASHD is a coronary angiogram, X-rays of the arteries of your heart. It is also the most formidable test. The decision as to whether you need a coronary angiogram should be made by your primary care physician and a cardiologist.

Doctors often have problems with patients admitted to a hospital with chest pain. They always seem to want to leave the next morning when they feel a little better. The diagnosis of a heart attack is usually very simple, *but it might take a couple of days!* When a piece of heart muscle dies, enzymes leak out of the dead and dying cells. These enzymes can be measured by blood tests. There are also usually characteristic changes in the EKG. It is not rare, however, for any or all of these tests to remain normal for as long as two days after your symptoms begin.

The treatment of angina has many facets. Any other condition that predisposes to ASHD must be eliminated if possible, and controlled if not. These include hypertension, diabetes, elevated blood levels of cholesterol and triglycerides, obesity, and smoking.

There are three basic kinds of medication for angina: nitrates, which come in all manner of pills, capsules, and patches; many different brands of beta blockers; and the newer calcium channel blockers. You may be given any one of them or all three.

Nitrates are nitrates. Whether you take a nitroglycerin under the tongue, swallow a pill or capsule, or wear a patch, they all do the same thing. The only differences are in the delivery method and duration of action. Nitrates are basically used for pain, for the symptomatic relief or prevention of angina. They cannot prevent a heart attack, and under most circumstances do not improve the health of your heart.

Beta blockers such as propranolol, the original, are a different story. They can prevent the symptoms of angina, but also have a tendency to sort of soothe the heart, to prevent abnormal electrical "rhythms" (see below), and they lower the blood pressure. They might, however, predispose to the development of congestive heart failure, which is discussed later, and cannot be taken if you suffer from asthma.

Calcium channel blockers are quite effective in preventing angina. They are thought to be particularly effective against vasospasm, and have the additional benefit of lowering the blood pressure.

Another form of treatment, for those most seriously afflicted, is coronary bypass surgery. There is some controversy over the indications to have such surgery. The most definite indication is if you are taking all the medication possible but still cannot live your life because of pain.

Dysrhythmias (also called arrhythmias) are another broad category of heart problems. The term literally means an abnormal rhythm. A dysrhythmia is an abnormal beating of the heart, either too slow (bradycardia), too fast (tachycardia), or irregularly. Most are caused by either a defect of the conducting system or an irritability of the heart muscle. A common word for the sensation of feeling a dysrhythmia is *palpitations*, but the sensing of palpitations has nothing at all to do with whether the dysrhythmia is of any significance or importance or not. As a matter of fact, *palpitations may be felt when there is no dysrhythmia at all!*

Most dysrhythmias are benign, of no real importance to the health of the individual. I would estimate that I see a hundred patients with benign dysrhythmias for every patient that has one of any significance.

Usually, it is only the sensation, the palpitation, that is the problem. A dysrhythmia can be serious if the heart is beating *excessively* fast or slow. A dysrhythmia can also be serious if it is indicative of an *excessive* irritability of the heart muscle. Let us look at some dysrhythmias, starting with defects in the conducting system.

Sometimes the SA node does not work normally, the "sick sinus syndrome." As mentioned previously, since the SA node under normal conditions will trigger a stimulus for the heart to beat faster than will any other part of the heart, it is the normal pacemaker. If it is not working properly, some other part of the heart will take over, but the heart will beat at a slower rate. There is more on this a little later.

The AV node can also fail to function normally. Sometimes it delays the stimulus from the atria to the ventricles too long. That is called first degree heart block, and it does not really cause a problem. Sometimes, some stimuli are blocked out altogether and the heart misses a beat, maybe every other, or every third one. That is called second degree heart block. It is not common, but when it exists, the heart is usually beating too slowly. Sometimes all stimuli are blocked completely. That is called third degree, or complete, heart block.

When stimuli from the SA node cannot reach the ventricles to make them contract, some other part of the heart will take over, and the heart will beat at a slower rate. Whether or not this causes any problems, symptoms, depends upon exactly how fast the heart does beat, and on the individual. If it is too slow, say forty times a minute or less, which is what commonly happens with complete heart block, the affected person may faint from insufficient blood reaching the brain, or go into congestive heart failure (described later) from lack of an adequate total cardiac output of blood.

Complete heart block is the most common (but not only) reason why artificial pacemakers are put into people. A pacemaker will electrically stimulate a heart to contract at a preset rate, usually seventy-two times per minute. Inserting a pacemaker used to involve surgery to open the chest cavity, to expose the heart. Now it has become a very simple procedure. The wire is inserted into the heart through a vein, and the battery is placed under the skin through a small incision.

Dysrhythmias that are due to an irritability of the heart muscle mostly fall into the category of premature contractions. There are two kinds, atrial and ventricular, and they are extremely common. These are what most patients mistakenly call skipped beats. When the heart beats before it is supposed to (before the next stimulus from the SA node arrives), there will be a longer than normal pause before the next contraction. The reason for this is that the arriving stimulus from the SA node will find a heart that has just contracted and is not ready to contract again. This longer pause gives the feeling of a skipped beat. Then, because the pause has allowed the heart to become filled with a greater than normal amount of blood, there will be a single harder than normal contraction, a thump.

Premature contractions can be eliminated with several different kinds of medication, but usually there is no medical need to do so. They are only of significance when there are many, many premature ventricular contractions per minute, or if they begin coming one right after another. Very often they are treated *only* because of a patient's fear of them, a reason I certainly consider to be a valid one. Let us look at some other common dysrhythmias.

There is a condition called paroxysmal atrial tachycardia that occurs usually in young women. It occurs in episodes, or paroxysms, hence the name. When this happens, the heart beats very fast, about one hundred sixty times a minute. Although it is a benign condition, it is a frightening one, and patients with it sometimes feel as if they are dying. It often can be stopped by pressing and rubbing on the carotid artery in the neck, or by taking a deep breath and pressing down hard, as if you were terribly constipated. If necessary, there is medication that will stop or prevent the attacks.

Ventricular tachycardia is another story entirely. This is an extremely serious dysrhythmia, fortunately relatively uncommon, that can lead to death. When it occurs, it is usually in conjunction with a heart attack.

Atrial fibrillation is a common dysrhythmia, and one of some importance. In this condition, the atria have lost the ability to contract as a unit. Instead, individual cells, or small bundles of cells, are contracting independently of each other. The atria feel like a bag of wiggling worms. Since the atria are not really pumping any blood into the ventricles, there is some loss of pumping efficiency on the part of the heart as a whole, but that is not usually very serious. The major problem with atrial fibrillation is that the AV node is constantly being bombarded with stimuli. Many, but not all, get through to the ventricles and make them beat too fast. Digoxin is usually used in this condition. It increases the block at the AV node, and allows the ventricles to beat at a normal rate.

Ventricular fibrillation is again a different story. When the ventricles fibrillate, the heart is not pumping any blood at all. That means death. This condition is a common reason for people to drop dead from a heart attack, often follows on the heel of ventricular tachycardia, and is the condition being treated when you see movies of the heart being given an electrical shock in an emergency room. *There is no connection between atrial fibrillation and ventricular fibrillation. One does not lead to the other.*

It is a common phenomenon for a patient to experience palpitations, and then come into the office and want an electrocardiogram, not understanding that *the EKG can only show the cause of the palpitations if the dysrhythmia occurs while the EKG is being taken.* There are two ways around this problem of "catching" the dysrhythmia on an EKG. You can wear a monitor for a day, that will continuously record your EKG. If your palpitations occur less frequently, you can rent a gadget that will enable you to transmit your EKG over the telephone whenever you experience palpitations.

There is one other, much less expensive, method of learning something about your palpitations. I often teach a patient, in whom I suspect nothing serious, how to check his own pulse rate. Many people experience a sensation of a rapid heart rate when they go to bed, and being able to confirm that their heart is beating normally is sometimes helpful in alleviating their fears.

We will look at some other, less common, heart problems. Myocarditis is an infection of the heart muscle usually caused by a virus. It fortunately is not very common, because sometimes the result is a heart too damaged to function properly.

A myocardopathy is a disease of heart muscle, and usually is a consequence of some other disease. Alcoholism is one of the more common causes, the combination of the alcohol and associated nutritional deficiencies leading to a weakened muscle that can cause heart failure and death.

Sometimes a virus can infect the pericardium. The term, as you might guess, is pericarditis. One possible complication of this disease is that the space between the pericardium and the heart can fill with fluid (a pericardial effusion) and impair the contraction of the heart. When that happens, the fluid must be drained out. Another complication occurs if the pericardium becomes scarred and contracted, again impairing the heart from pumping properly. Surgery alleviates this condition if necessary.

Congestive heart failure is an extremely common heart condition. It comes about when the heart is not working optimally as a pump. *Congestive heart failure is not a disease. It is a condition that is always caused by some underlying disease.* The net result of congestive heart failure is the accumulation of salt and water in the body. This water settles either in the lungs, causing shortness of breath, or in the legs, causing edema, or in both. The word *failure* has an ominous sound to it, as if death were imminent, but that is not usually the case. People can go on for years, decades, with congestive heart failure, if they take care of themselves. The extreme form of congestive heart failure is called pulmonary edema, and that can quickly lead to death.

The treatment of congestive heart failure may be directed at the heart disease itself, but more commonly it is aimed at helping the heart and kidneys get rid of the accumulated salt and water. Sometimes the cause of the congestive heart failure is a dysrhythmia. Control of the heart rate in these cases is critical. Drinking less fluids may seem to be a logical treatment, but it usually is not. Water goes where the salt is, so elimination of salt from the diet is obviously the first step. Diuretics are an important medication for this condition. Many patients will take a form of digitalis, such as digoxin, which makes the heart beat more strongly and leads to an increased formation of urine.

CHAPTER 15

THE LUNGS

Everyone knows that the lungs are in the chest, but many people do not realize how big they are. They extend from front to back, and from near the bottom edge of the rib cage all the way up to the space between the shoulder and neck. Indeed, aside from the esophagus, the great blood vessels, and the relatively small heart and the tissues it sits in, there is nothing else in the chest but lung. To picture the pulmonary system, imagine an upside-down tree almost completely imbedded in an enormous sponge. The trunk is the trachea, or windpipe; the branches are the bronchi; and the sponge is the lung tissue itself, millions of little air pockets called alveoli.

The lungs are what nature has developed for us to exchange gases, oxygen and carbon dioxide, with the atmosphere. When life was just one cell, or a few cells, floating in a prehistoric ocean, it was simple for dissolved gases to pass between the water and the inside of the cells. Such passive diffusion of gas, however, could not supply the needs of larger animals. An organ to speed up the process was necessary. Fish developed gills. Land animals need lungs. With each breath, oxygen in the air is taken into the blood in the lungs, and carbon dioxide (the end product of the burning of our sugar fuel) is released.

The most common medical problems of this respiratory system involve infections, difficulty in breathing or shortness of breath, blood

117

clots, and tumors. We will discuss them, but first, let us understand a little about coughing.

Coughing is caused by an irritation within the lungs. It is a reflex, designed to expel unwanted material. Sometimes a relative of an old, weak, debilitated patient will ask me when I think the person will pass away. Often my answer is: "When he's too weak to cough." Coughing keeps us alive. Our lungs are exposed to everything and anything in the air, and that includes dust, dirt, fumes, and germs of an almost infinite variety. There are several mechanisms that either filter out or propel out these unwanted invaders, but the act of last resort is the cough. Without the cough, anything we inhaled by accident (as when something we are supposed to swallow goes down the wrong pipe) would remain in the lungs forever, and the slightest infection would lead to death. I am belaboring this point because so many patients seem to think that the cough medicine I presecribe is supposed to stop them from coughing completely, or even is supposed to make their cold go away. Neither of those beliefs is true. The purpose of most cough medicines is twofold, to help liquify the phlegm so that it can be coughed out of the lungs more easily, and to take the "edge" off the coughing, to make it more tolerable. Without coughing, chest colds would become fatal cases of pneumonia. Now do not worry about that and be afraid to take cough medicines! They are not strong enough to completely stop a necessary cough!

With our discussion of infections, we will start at the top of the pulmonary tree and work our way down.

Infections of the trachea are more of a problem in the pediatric age group. Adults experience tracheitis as part of a chest cold. That is the raw sensation you feel in the front of your chest when you breathe.

Bronchitis is, by far, the most common pulmonary infection. There are two basic types, acute and chronic.

On several occasions I have had patients tell me that they have suffered with bronchitis, their tone implying that they had some serious kind of pulmonary ailment. Likewise, sometimes when a diagnosis of acute bronchitis has been put on an insurance form, the patient has reacted as if he had been told that he has some dread disease.

Understand that the medical term for a chest cold is "acute bronchitis." They are synonymous. Chronic bronchitis is something else entirely.

Most cases of acute bronchitis are caused by either viruses or bacteria, but it is not uncommon for a chest cold to begin as a viral infection and then become a bacterial one. Many people do not like going to doctors, and there is nothing wrong with treating yourself for a chest cold with cough medicine, rest, plenty of fluids, and a vaporizer (the cold-mist type puts more moisture into the air) if it is winter and the air inside is dry. But be reasonable about it! If you feel very weak and sick, you might have pneumonia. Do not treat yourself without seeing a doctor for more than a reasonable period of time. If you are not feeling better, if the cough and/or fever is not subsiding after several days, see your doctor.

Patients who do see a physician for a chest cold will often be given a prescription for an antibiotic. The necessity for antibiotics in this condition is not always certain. Sometimes I prescribe them, sometimes I do not. Remember, if the infecting agent is a virus, the antibiotic will do nothing. If you do take antibiotics, however, the best way to know that it is working, and this holds true for any lung infection, is to pay attention to the color of your sputum, the phlegm that you bring up when you cough. A definite lightening of the color after a few days means that the infection is subsiding. *The cough itself, however, is going to take much, much longer to go away.*

Chronic bronchitis is a smouldering infection due to a degenerative disease of the bronchi. Affected patients cough up phlegm almost every day, and acute flare-ups are common. The treatment of chronic bronchitis involves the stopping of smoking (a usual causative factor), vaporizers, and medications to open the bronchi and help clean out the infected material. Antibiotics are used for the episodes of acute infection, and some physicians prescribe them periodically to treat the underlying disease. Emphysema is a common consequence of chronic bronchitis. We will discuss that condition after the next paragraph.

Some patients develop wheezing when they have a chest cold. This condition is called asthmatic bronchitis, and should not be confused with true asthma. In both cases, however, the wheezing is caused by constriction of the bronchi. This narrows the air passages, making it difficult to move air primarily out of the lungs. The treatment of asthmatic bronchitis is the same as acute bronchitis except for the addition of asthma-type medication, which helps expand and open the bronchi. True asthma is not caused by an infection, and in the more severe cases requires treatment by lung specialists.

Emphysema is a condition where the very thin membranous walls between the microscopic air pockets of the lungs break down. These walls are where the oxygen you breathe in gets into your blood, and the carbon dioxide you manufacture gets out of you into the air. When too much of this tissue disappears, you simply do not have enough lung to breathe with. Chronic bronchitis is by no means the only way to develop emphysema, although it is among the most common, but whatever the reason, the damage done by emphysema is permanent and irreversible.

Bronchiectasis is a condition where the wall of the bronchus has broken down. The result is a sack of infected material that cannot be helped much by antibiotics. Surgery to remove the affected section of lung is the only cure in severe cases.

Pneumonia is a more severe kind of pulmonary infection. In these cases it is the alveoli themselves that are infected. There are various forms of pneumonia, some affecting an entire lobe of a lung, some just a segment of a lobe. Like acute bronchitis, pneumonia can also be viral or bacterial, or in some cases caused by other kinds of infecting organisms. Although it is certainly possible to recover from pneumonia without medical treatment, that approach is a foolhardy risk of life. If you do get true pneumonia, do not expect to feel yourself again for at least a month and a half.

Patients with pneumonia always seem anxious to know what their latest chest X-ray shows. The fact is that improvement in the chest X-ray lags far behind the actual improvement in the patient by many days, or even weeks.

Perhaps the most severe form of lung infection is a pulmonary abscess. In pneumonia, the basic structure of the lung is usually preserved. With an abscess, the infected part of the lung is destroyed, leaving a pus-filled cavity. Lung abscesses usually occur in people who are for one reason or another debilitated and prone to infections. Surgery is sometimes necessary to save the patient's life.

For some reason I do not understand, many patients who are given antibiotics for a lung infection do not take them for the prescribed length of time. Do not be one of them. Your doctor writes the number of pills or capsules he wants you to take on the prescription. Take them all.

Pulmonary embolization is one of the most insidious lung diseases. An embolus, as noted earlier, is a clot that forms in a blood vessel, either an artery or a vein (or the heart), then breaks free, traveling with the blood until it gets lodged in a small artery. A pulmonary embolus forms in a large vein in the leg or pelvis, then breaks free, travels through the great veins, through the right side of the heart, then lodges in a pulmonary artery in the lung. The clot blocks the flow of blood to that section of the lung, the size of the area involved depending upon the size of the clot. Often, if the clot is large enough, and the outer lining of the lung is involved, it will also cause a great deal of pain, but sometimes that is not the case. Often there will be phlebitis pain where the clot has formed, but many times there is little or no pain there either. As stated in an earlier chapter, if a clot does form in a large vein, the less pain it causes, the more likely it is that it will break loose and become an embolus. Tests to determine if a patient has had a pulmonary embolus (a lung scan and arterial blood gases are the most common) are not very sensitive, especially if the embolus is small. These are the many reasons why a pulmonary embolus, or even many small emboli, often go undiagnosed by the most competent physician. Even when suspected, it is often impossible to prove that it has happened. Physicians nevertheless sometimes treat their patient on the basis of suspicion alone because the next embolus may be a large, and fatal, one.

A somewhat typical case would be the young woman who came to my office complaining of a slight pain she had on the side of her chest for a few days. She had felt a little short of breath, but that was subsiding, as was the chest pain. As matter of fact, she had almost canceled her appointment. I asked her if she had any leg or calf pain. She denied it. I examined her, finding nothing at all wrong, except for perhaps the barest discomfort when I squeezed one of her calves. I was just about ready at that point to conclude that there was probably nothing much wrong with her when she recalled that she did have some pain in her calf about two weeks earlier, that she had even limped a little for a few days. I have never considered it my business to take chances with someone else's health or life. I hospitalized her and began treating her with an anticoagulant. In her case, the subsequent lung scan showed the embolus. It often does not. Without that, I still would not know for certain if she had one or not.

Many people mistakenly believe that the anticoagulant medication used to treat a pulmonary embolus will dissolve the clot. That is not the case. There are such dissolving medications, but they have potentially serious side effects, which make their use risky. In most cases they are not really necessary. The blood contains natural enzymes that will, in time, dissolve the clot. In those uncommon instances of a truly massive pulmonary embolus, emergency surgery to remove it is necessary. The treatment of a pulmonary embolus is aimed at preventing more of them, and is the treatment for acute deep vein thrombophlebitis as outlined in Chapter 13. The one difference may be that the patient will take oral anticoagulants for a longer period of time.

There are many kinds of malignant tumors, cancers, of the lung, and they are a depressing group of diseases. There is no sure way to detect them early, and available treatment is not very satisfactory. Unfortunately, a lung tumor has to be quite sizeable before it can be seen on a chest X-ray, and by that time it has usually already spread. Some people are cured, however. Surgical removal, when that is possible, and cobalt radiation are the usual treatments.

Shortness of breath (the medical term for this is dyspnea, as noted earlier) is such a common complaint of patients that I am including this section to give you a bird's-eye view of that symptom.

The more common lung diseases or conditions that can cause dyspnea include serious infections such as pneumonia, asthma or asthmatic bronchitis, emphysema, replacement of lung tissue with tumor, congestive heart failure as described in the chapter on the heart, and large or multiple pulmonary emboli.

Sometimes dyspnea is due to what is called a pleural effusion. This is a condition where fluid collects inside the chest cavity, but outside the lungs. If there is enough fluid, it compresses the lung and makes breathing difficult. There are many causes of pleural effusions. They include infections, malignancies, and congestive heart failure.

Sometimes people display a lack of simple common sense. Many times patients coming to me complaining about their shortness of breath (and they are usually convinced they have a fatal heart or lung disease) will state that they have little or no difficulty with their breathing when they are walking, or even exercising. They usually feel their symptoms when relatively inactive. It should be obvious that if any "physical" problem with the heart or lungs is severe enough to cause dyspnea at rest, exercise would be next to impossible. That brings us again to the most common cause of shortness of breath, by far, and it has nothing at all to do with the lungs or heart. As mentioned earlier, it is the result of common anxiety, and is called the hyperventilation syndrome. It is discussed more fully in Chapter 22.

CHAPTER 16

EDEMA

Edema is the abnormal retention of water in the tissues, usually the legs and ankles. In other words, I am talking about swollen feet and legs. As with anemia and congestive heart failure, edema is a condition, not a disease. It is always caused by something else. Edema is such a common problem, and causes so many to have discomfort and complications, and so few people take care of it properly, that I decided to devote a chapter to it.

There are really two kinds of edema. One kind is called nonpitting edema. It is due to an obstruction to the flow of lymph, and is so rare I will say no more about it. The usual kind is pitting edema, so called because if you press on it, your fingertip will leave a hole or pit. You can check yourself for edema. Find the flat surface of bone on the inside front of your lower leg, just above your ankle. Press in firmly with your fingertip for a couple of seconds, then remove it. Do you see or feel a hole? If there is more than the slightest depression, you have some edema.

Why is edema important? One reason is that it can be indicative of a serious disease. The more common reason, however, is because if you have a significant amount of edema, and do not take care of it, you are likely to suffer the complications, aside from having to carry around the five to ten pounds, or more, of extra weight in your legs all day! Think about that a moment if you think you get tired too easily!

How does edema form? A small amount of fluid normally exists between all the cells of your body. This intercellular fluid is salt water that is constantly oozing out of the small arteries, and is constantly being absorbed back into the blood by the small veins. There are many factors controlling the rates at which this fluid is being formed and removed. They include the pressure of the blood in the smallest arteries, the pressure of the blood in the veins, the total amount of salt and water in the body, and the amount of a protein, albumin, in the blood.

Why does edema so commonly affect the lower legs and ankles instead of other parts of the body? The answer is simple. Gravity. Water runs downhill to the lowest level. Indeed, patients prone to edema who are confined in bed for prolonged periods will develop sacral edema in the lower back.

Some of the conditions that can cause edema are serious. Congestive heart failure, which is discussed in the chapter on the heart, severe liver disease, and severe kidney disease, all cause the body to retain salt and water. An obstruction to the flow of blood in the veins, such as a tumor or a clot, will raise the pressure of the blood in the veins and prevent the intercellular fluid from being absorbed back into the blood. Some patients who are malnourished, or who lose a lot of protein in the urine, will have lower than normal amounts of albumin in the blood, and develop edema. The most common cause of edema, however, is varicosities of the big veins in the legs as described in Chapter 13. As with an obstruction, the increased pressure of the blood in the leg veins prevents the normal absorption of the intercellular fluid, and it simply accumulates and becomes edema. Since the most common cause of varicosities is pregnancy, women suffer from chronic edema more than men. If in addition to having this kind of problem with veins, you also have even a minimal problem with your heart, or kidneys, or liver, the amount of edema will be increased.

The common complications of chronic significant edema are cellulitis and ulcers of the legs. Cellulitis, as already noted, is an infection of the skin. It can cause severe pain, very high fever, and often requires hospitalization. A small minor infection can spread rapidly in edematous tissues. If you can picture the difference in the strength between paper that is dry and paper that is soaking wet, you will have an idea of what chronic edema does to the strength and resistance of your skin. Chronically edematous skin is easily damaged. Germs get in and grow well in all that water inside. Sometimes the area of infection is localized and you get an ulcer, and sometimes the infection spreads and you get cellulitis. Sometimes the skin becomes chronically infected and inflamed; that is called stasis dermatitis.

Phlebitis, inflammation of veins with clots in them, is another possible complication of chronic edema. This problem is discussed in the chapter on the vascular system.

The treatment of edema must first be aimed at any serious condition causing or contributing to it. If none of those are present, then the following is in order.

Eliminate all excess salt from your diet. Where salt goes, so goes water, and the less salt you have in your body, the less water you will have also. If salt restriction is not enough, and it may not be, a diuretic will help.

I tell my patients to spend forty-five minutes, three times a day, lying on their back with their feet higher than their head. This empties the veins of all that blood, decreases the pressure inside the veins to almost zero, and allows the excess water in the legs to be absorbed into the veins, eventually to be urinated out. That is why you will probably notice that your legs are least swollen in the morning and most swollen at night. As noted, it all has to do with gravity. Advice such as this often seems to fall on deaf ears. I have had the experience on many occasions of hospitalizing a patient who is chronically edematous and finding that their edema disappears in a day or two. It becomes obvious, and annoying, that they have been ignoring my suggestions all along.

Snug surgical-type stockings can help in the prevention of edema. The compressing pressure helps force fluid into the veins and out of your legs. But be careful that you do not allow the tops of the stockings to become tight bands! That can hurt more than it helps!

If you have developed a degree of cellulitis, *superficial* phlebitis, or an ulcer, add the treatment of a wet heating pad during the time you are on your back with your legs up. The heat will help heal the inflammation or infection.

I have one more thought to add to all of the above. I think it is quite likely that a large excess of abdominal fat can contribute to the formation of edema in the legs. All those pounds can press on the big veins in the abdomen and prevent the easy escape of blood from the legs. So that is another reason to lose weight.

CHAPTER 17

HYPERTENSION

Hypertension means high blood pressure; the terms are synonymous. Hypertension is one of the commonest afflictions in our society. It is an insidious disease, usually producing no symptoms until it is too late. You can feel terrific, in the pink, robust and hearty, but all the while your body is suffering ongoing irreparable damage. Many people seem to make much of the fact that high blood pressure can cause headaches, assuming that since they do not suffer from headaches their blood pressure must be okay. Nothing could be further from the truth. *During eighteeen years of practicing medicine, I have had only three or four patients with headaches due to hypertension!*

There is a much more common relationship between high blood pressure and headaches. Emotional tension and stress are common accompaniments of hypertension, so it is not unusual for patients to have hypertension and tension headaches at the same time, but the headaches do not go away when the blood pressure is brought down to normal, *and having the headache does not mean that your pressure is high*. I have one patient whose blood pressure is under excellent control with medication, yet every time she gets a headache she thinks it is due to her pressure and comes in to have it checked. I cannot seem to convince her that the two are not related.

Most people are mystified by how a blood pressure is taken, and what the numbers mean, but it is not difficult to understand, so let us start with that. Let us imagine a boy who is trying hard to fill his soft, leaky bicycle tire with a hand pump. Each time he pushes down on the pump, he pumps air into the tire. The pressure inside the tire rises and it swells a little. But while he is raising the pump handle for another downstroke, the air is leaking out. The tire is slowly deflating and the air pressure inside is falling. But the boy is full of energy, and the leak in the tire is small, so the pressure in the tire does not fall to zero before he pumps more air into it. We can picture him on his knees, forever pumping the air in, and hearing it leak out, the tire expanding and contracting in rhythm with his efforts, the pressure inside reaching a peak, and then a valley. That is the exact situation with blood pressure. The heart is the pump, the tire represents your arteries, and the air leaking out is the blood flowing out of the arteries into the veins. If the boy attached a tube from the leak to his hand pump, so that he was continually reusing the same air, we would have a truly identical situation. When the heart contracts it propels blood into the arteries, expanding them a little, raising the pressure inside to a peak. After the heart contracts, it relaxes and fills with blood before contracting again. During this time, some of the blood in the arteries is flowing into the veins, and the pressure inside the arteries is falling. The two numbers of a blood pressure reading represent the measurement of these highs and lows, written as a fraction with the highest pressure over the lowest pressure.

It is also not hard to understand how the blood pressure is measured. When your doctor inflates the blood pressure cuff, it is so tight that it completely stops the flow of blood into your lower arm. He then slowly lets the air out, listening with his stethescope over the artery, while watching the falling blood pressure gauge. When the point is reached that the pressure in the cuff is low enough to allow the blood to get past at its peak pressure (immediately after a heart contraction), a spurt of blood shoots through, and makes a sound that he hears. That is the highest, or *systolic* pressure. As he continues to listen, he hears more spurts because the cuff is still not allowing blood to get past while the heart is relaxed. Finally, the spurts stop. The blood is flowing smoothly again because even the lowest pressure in the arteries is enough to force blood past the cuff. That is the lowest, or *diastolic* pressure.

When doctors use the term hypertension, they really mean "essential hypertension," and that is defined as having a constantly elevated *diastolic* pressure. When the systolic pressure is too high, it is called systolic hypertension. When the blood pressure is too high only at certain times, it is called labile hypertension. Finally, when someone has high blood pressure because of some known reason, such as certain kidney diseases, or tumors that secrete certain hormones in excess, it is called secondary hypertension. Systolic hypertension is mostly an effect of the aging process, and, unless severe, does not have to be treated. We will discuss essential hypertension (calling it simply "hypertension") and labile hypertension, which, except in extreme or unusual circumstances, is not really a disease at all.

What are the long-term consequences of uncontrolled hypertension? The effects are on the heart and arteries. The blood pressure is created and maintained by the contractions of the heart. Obviously, if the heart is forced to keep blood flowing at a higher than normal pressure, it has to be working harder. Hypertensive heart disease is a condition where the heart becomes enlarged, and the muscular wall thickened. Eventually the heart becomes unable to maintain the pressure and begins to fail.

Arteries that are forced to endure an excessive pressure inside them also become thickened, and, in the process, narrowed. What we have is a rapid acceleration of arteriosclerotic disease. The arteries most seriously affected are those inside the kidneys, the brain, and the coronary arteries in the heart. Nephrosclerosis is the kidney disease caused by high blood pressure. It can destroy the kidneys completely. The effects of hypertension on the brain and heart lead to strokes and heart attacks. Remember, most of the damage done to these vital organs by high blood pressure is irreversible, permanent. It will not be pleasant if you are told that you have high blood pressure after a stroke leaves you half paralyzed, or you have a heart attack and cannot work anymore, or your kidneys are so damaged that you have to spend the rest of your life using a dialysis machine. Get your pressure checked. If it is high, take the medication as you are told to take it.

There are dozens of different kinds of medication for hypertension. They work in many, many different ways, and each has its own potential side effects. Diuretics are commonly used. The removal of some salt water from the body lowers the blood pressure significantly. Often, some other kind of blood pressure medication will be prescribed in addition to the water pills. Every physician has his favorites. There are two fundamental truths, however. You should stay away from salt, and the blood pressure medication *will only work while it is in your body!*

I have to expand on the above a little. Too often I have placed patients with hypertension on medication, checked them soon thereafter to make certain that their pressure had come down to normal, and then had the experience of not seeing them for years. When they do return, they are not on their medication. "Why?" I ask.

"I had it checked," they reply with a shrug. "It was normal, so I stopped taking the pills."

The facts of the matter are that you can take the medication every day for ten years, having normal blood pressure all the time, yet a couple of days after you stop taking it you will have high blood pressure again. Let us say it once more. *The medicine only works while it is in your body. There are no beneficial aftereffects if you stop taking it.*

What should you do if you are told that your pressure is borderline? First of all, remember that blood pressure tends to rise as you get older. If a borderline blood pressure is your only problem, the answer is to lose some weight, stay away from salt, and have your pressure checked regularly. If you also have diabetes, a borderline blood pressure is more important. Both diseases have long-term adverse effects on the arteries, and the effects can be additive. I believe that diabetics with borderline hypertension should be treated so that they have absolutely normal blood pressure.

That brings us to the question of how often you need to have your blood pressure checked. Not that often! If it has been normal, I mentioned in Chapter 2 approximately how often people should have routine checkups. As deadly as hypertension can be, it does need a lot of time, many, many years, to work its damage. If you have hypertension, you will have to be checked more often. Certainly, during the time it is being brought under control with medication, you may have to visit the doctor as often as every week. Once it has been brought down to normal, however, I see my patients with hypertension just two to four times a year. I do not believe more frequent visits are necessary. Fixed hypertension rarely changes drastically over a short period of time. A new patient once told me he had been seeing a doctor to have his pressure checked two to four times a month for over a year! Except for highly unusual circumstances, that is a rip-off.

I personally have encountered little difficulty in convincing my patients to stay on the antihypertensive medication I prescribe, at least not in recent years. I make certain that they understand that they have to take their medication forever, and I do not hesitate to scare them a little with the truth, as I have tried to do to you. I have, however, had great difficulty, on occasion, convincing new patients that they *do not* have high blood pressure! That brings us to the subject of labile (changing) hypertension.

Blood pressure is anything but stable. It varies almost constantly, depending upon our physical activity and emotions. It can be high in many, many people under conditions that cause stress and anxiety, *such as being in a doctor's office and having their blood pressure checked.* The point here is that one high blood pressure reading or even two may be meaningless. This is especially true if it is a first visit to a new doctor. When I find an elevated blood pressure reading, I always have the patient rest quietly after the examination and tests are completed, preferably reading a magazine to get his mind off where he is, and then measure his pressure again, and a third and fourth time if necessary. Only then, if the reading remains elevated, am I satisfied that he really does have hypertension.

There are occasional extreme cases of labile hypertension, especially in those with sensitive and volatile cardiovascular systems who are subject to intense emotional pressures. Some patients with more severe forms may, at some point in the future, even develop fixed hypertension. That is a reason for a periodic checkup. There are those in the medical community, however, who have recently begun to try to expand the scope and importance of labile hypertension to the point that they are almost calling a normal physiologic reaction (what has historically been called the "fight or flight mechanism") a disease. That, of course, is as ridiculous as the faddish hypoglycemia explosion of a few years ago.

Many physicians, very incorrectly I believe, treat patients with transient stress-induced labile hypertension. I would estimate that I personally would have three times as many patients on medication, medication they do not need, if I relied on the first blood pressure reading alone. So it is not an unusual situation, when patients come to me for the first time with a history of having had high blood pressure for any number of years, that when I check their pressure for the third or fourth time I find readings at the *low* range of normal! Usually, the medication they have been taking is minimal and could not possibly account for it. When I ask them how many times their doctor had checked their pressure during each visit, they invariably answer once. I explain the situation, and the concept of labile hypertension, to them, but you would be surprised how difficult it is to convince them that they do not have high blood pressure, and probably never did! Some have even decided that I must be a quack and have never come back!

In summary, do not accept a diagnosis of hypertension unless your pressure is checked after you have had a chance to relax a while. Do not commit yourself to taking medication for the rest of your life unless the disease is really present.

CHAPTER 18

THE GASTROINTESTINAL TRACT

The gastrointestinal tract begins with the mouth, ends with the anus, and includes the esophagus, which is the tube connecting the mouth to the stomach, the stomach, the small and large intestines, and the associated organs, the liver, gall bladder, and pancreas. We will begin with a very few words about the mouth and work our way down.

The mouth receives the food, and the teeth are meant to chew it *into a semisolid before it is swallowed!* More on that later. The swallowed food passes through the esophagus and enters the stomach. There is normally a valve of sorts at the junction of the esophagus and stomach that prevents food from leaving the stomach in the wrong direction. (Remember our earlier discussion of the words *stomach* and *abdomen*. The abdomen is the entire area between the diaphragm and pelvis, between just above the lowest ribs to just above the groin. The stomach is a relatively small pouch that receives and holds the swallowed food. It is located in the "pit" of the abdomen, that soft area in the center of the upper abdomen.) One of the major functions of the stomach is to secrete an acid that mixes with the food to help in digestion. From the stomach, the food passes into the very long small intestine. The first portion of the small intestine is called the duodenum.

The esophagus, stomach, and duodenum constitute what is called the upper G.I. tract. Many of the more common problems of this area are caused by the acid that is produced in the stomach. It can cause what amounts to a chemical burn, an irritation and inflammation of the esophagus (esophagitis), the stomach itself (gastritis), or the duodenum (duodenitis).

Esophagitis causes a burning pain in the mid and lower chest called heartburn. Gastritis and duodenitis cause pain or discomfort in the pit of the abdomen. There also may be a feeling of stuffiness or indigestion, and belching and excess gas. There is a way to distinguish between an inflamed stomach and an inflamed duodenum. If eating bland food makes you feel a little worse, the problem is probably in your stomach. If it makes you feel better, the problem is probably in your duodenum. If the pain is intense, bores through into your back, or wakes you up at night, you probably have progressed to the point of having an ulcer, so let us discuss ulcers.

There are basically two kinds of ulcers, the common duodenal, and the less common stomach, or gastric. An ulcer is simply an erosion in the internal lining of the area involved. A duodenal ulcer classically causes a severe pain in the pit of the stomach that often penetrates through to the back. It characteristically feels better after eating bland food, and often causes enough pain at night to wake the sufferer up. There are three common complications of duodenal ulcers, if they are not properly treated. The ulcer can eat its way through the wall of the duodenum and either penetrate into the pancreas behind it, or into the abdominal cavity. The latter requires surgery. It can erode into a blood vessel and begin to bleed, sometimes quite massively. Finally, a chronic ulcer can cause enough inflammation and scarring to obstruct the emptying of the stomach, a condition again requiring surgery.

There is another kind of problem with a gastric ulcer. Sometimes it forms in a malignancy, and X-rays cannot reliably differentiate between a so-called benign gastric ulcer and a malignant one. Care of a gastric ulcer used to involve repeated X-ray procedures to make certain that it healed and did not recur. Now, the area can be biopsied with a gastroscope to see if any cancer is present, although that is not always foolproof either.

Under usual circumstances, these above conditions do not arise unless the area is challenged with a greater than normal amount of acid secretion and/or with foods that are themselves acid, although there are probably other factors involved in the development of an ulcer. Coffee, tea, chocolate, and colas contain caffeine or other chemicals that increase the secretion of stomach acid. Carbonated beverages and most fruit juices are themselves acid. Tobacco, alcohol, aspirin, other medications, many spices, and emotional stress add to the problem.

There are two basic tests for this region of the body. An upper G.I. series is an X-ray study performed after swallowing barium that will show the esophagus, stomach, and duodenum. (It will not, as many people assume, show the gall bladder.) A gastroscopy will allow a physician to directly see the same area. As I have stated previously, I do not believe in jumping to do these tests unless symptoms are very severe, or my patient has not responded to treatment in a reasonable period of time.

The treatment for all the above conditions is basically the same with some variations. Avoid all foods that are acid or that increase the secretion of acid, take antacids, and, if necessary, a medication that decreases the secretion of acid, and/or a medication that coats and protects the ulcer. A word more about antacids. Often, a patient who complains to me about symptoms such as the above will also have correctly diagnosed his problem, but then tell me that he took an antacid once or twice with little benefit. Remember, acid is being secreted almost constantly, and the inflammation will take some time to subside even after all acid is neutralized. The key to feeling better, and getting better, is *frequency* of antacid administration. A teaspoon or two every hour or two is far better than a glassful twice a day. And remember what I said about the difference between feeling better and healing, between treating symptoms and treating the disease. To be certain that everything is healed, you have to continue the therapy for some time after all symptoms subside. Otherwise you are likely to have a quick recurrence of your discomfort. In some patients with chronic problems, antacids and other medications have to be taken for extended periods of time.

We will discuss three other problems of the upper G.I. tract. The most common of these is a hiatus hernia, a condition many people have heard about, but few seem to understand.

The stomach is normally entirely within the abdomen. When a

portion of the stomach works its way through the diaphragm into the lower chest, it is called a hiatus hernia.

A hiatus hernia can cause problems two basic ways. If you will recall, there is a valve of sorts at the junction of the esophagus and stomach that prevents food from going back up. That valve may stop working when you have a hiatus hernia. The contents of the stomach can then freely move up into the esophagus, especially when you lie down, and cause an almost continuous "reflux" esophagitis. The key to treatment is to not eat before going to bed, and to take a lot of antacid. Sometimes it may be necessary to take the medication I mentioned above to decrease the secretion of acid.

The other problem of a hiatus hernia is that a large bubble of gas can become trapped in the hernia pouch that is itself trapped above the diaphragm. That can cause pressure symptoms in the chest mimicking heart pain. The best way to deal with this is to avoid swallowing air, and to use an over-the-counter medication called simethicone to help belch up the gas. There is more on this problem of gas later.

Some people develop a condition called pylorospasm, a painful tightening, or spasm, in the pit of the abdomen that may not be responsive to the antacid therapy outlined above. Addition of antispasmodics often helps in these cases.

Some people have a problem with their stomach in that it will not empty normally. The food just lies there and they feel very uncomfortable. There is a fairly new prescription medication available that may help certain patients with this condition quite dramatically. I recall one man who came to me with a ten-year history of having very uncomfortable stomach symptoms after eating. His symptoms disappeared almost overnight with that medication. It did cause a problem on one occasion, however. I prescribed it for a patient who went to have an upper G.I. series a few days later. The medication worked so well that the radiologist could not do the procedure! The barium would not stay in the stomach!

The small intestine is very long, and is where food is digested and absorbed into the blood. Digestion is actually only a chemical breakdown of food into its basic components. This is accomplished by a host of enzymes that are secreted into the small intestine by the pancreas and glands lining the wall of the small intestine itself. Fat, since it does not mix with water, requires something else for its digestion, bile. Bile is an emulsifier, allowing fat to sort of dissolve in water. There will be more on bile later.

Diseases of the small intestine are relatively uncommon. Tumors are rare. Perhaps the most common disease is an inflammatory condition of the end of the small intestine called regional ileitis, or regional enteritis. In its mild forms, treatment with medication is very helpful. In its severe forms it can be devastating.

Some people develop any one of a number of conditions that lead to a malabsorption syndrome, an inability to properly digest one kind of food or another. Symptoms are usually weight loss and severe diarrhea. Fortunately, the more severe types of these conditions are fairly uncommon. There are some people, however, who develop an intolerance to milk sugar (latose), or to grain products. If you are having a problem with persistent cramps and diarrhea, it is worth the effort to eliminate one, and then the other, of these foods for a time to see if your symptoms are relieved.

The small intestine empties into the large intestine, or colon. Here water is removed from the intestinal contents and a stool is formed. The very end of the colon is called the rectum, and the opening the stool passes out through is called the anus. The anus, rectum, and colon constitute the lower G.I. tract.

Probably the most common problem with this part of the body is hemorrhoids. These are nothing more than varicose veins of the anus. There are two basic kinds, the external, which can hurt, but less commonly bleed, and the internal, which can bleed, but cannot hurt. Treatments include agents that soften and lubricate the stool, wet heat, and over-the-counter creams. Excessive bleeding from internal hemorrhoids is often treated by putting small rubber bands around them. They clot and eventually fall off. Excessive problems with external hemorrhoids require surgery.

Many of the diseases of the lower G.I. tract manifest themselves with the symptoms of cramps and diarrhea, and there are a host of them. Many different kinds of microorganisms can cause infections in the colon. Cholera is perhaps the worst of these, affecting the entire intestine. Bacillary and amebic dysentery are also severe infectious diseases. They are usually transmitted by improper handling of sewage. (By the way, do not use the word *dysentery* if what you mean is *diarrhea*.) The most common infecting organisms of the colon that we have to deal with, however, are viruses, although there are other organisms that cause problems on occasion.

As with the small intestine, there are inflammatory diseases of the colon. The most severe is ulcerative colitis. In this disorder, the inner lining of the colon becomes very inflamed and ulcerated, even sometimes to the point of bleeding profusely. Milder cases can respond very well to treatment with medications. The more severe forms of the disease sometimes require removal of the large intestine.

The most common cause of chronic cramps and diarrhea is not a disease, but a functional disorder called a spastic colon, or irritable bowel syndrome. The term *functional* implies that the colon is not diseased, just overactive. If you have persistent cramps and diarrhea, but have no fever, are eating normally, see no blood in the stool, and otherwise feel healthy, that is probably what you have, but have it checked by a doctor. This condition can be very difficult, if not impossible, to treat. Potent antispasmodics often do very little. Patients suffering from it frequently keep asking about, and searching for, a proper diet. It has been my experience that diet seldom makes any difference if it is really a spastic colon, and if it does, the improvement is only temporary. The condition is mentioned again in the chapter dealing with psychosomatic disorders.

Diverticulosis and diverticulitis are very common problems. Remember, *-osis* means you have them, *-itis* means that one or more are infected. A single diverticulum is a small pouch protruding out of the colon. If you can picture removing a small circle of rubber from a tire with an inner tube, and seeing the inner tube ballooning out, that is a diverticulum. They tend to form in that part of the colon nearest the rectum. Most of the time there are many, perhaps many dozen. They can cause alternating constipation and diarrhea, and sometimes the leakage of liquid stool from the anus. For the latter condition I recommend small doses of over-the-counter medication containing kaolin and pectin, which can soak up the excess water. The major problem with diverticulosis is developing diverticulitis. That usually happens when the opening of one of the pouches becomes clogged and an infection develops. In the extreme, the infection can progress to a true abscess and require surgery. Most of the time, however, the infection responds to antibiotics. If you have diverticulosis, the best way to prevent such an infection from developing is to stay completely away from seeds and nuts, indigestible particles that can block the openings to the diverticula. Remember, that includes corn, tomatoes and cucumbers, unless you remove the seeds, and seeded bread and rolls.

The usual tests for the colon are the barium enema, an X-ray examination, and the various endoscopic procedures outlined in the chapter on tests.

Constipation is one of the most common complaints I hear, especially from the elderly. Constipation really means excessively hard stools. The word for an inability to move the bowels is *obstipation*. Since every patient uses the word constipation to mean obstipation, however, I will also.

Many people complaining about constipation do not really have it at all. What they suffer from is the unreasonable expectation of moving their bowels every day. It is not abnormal to move your bowels every other day, or every third day, or sometimes even every fourth day, as long as the bowel movement is normal, not excessively hard. If hard stools are your problem, take an over-the-counter stool softener. Many patients will tell me that they took one a day for a few days and it did not help. That is not surprising. You have to take enough, and for a long enough period of time, for it to work. If the problem is that you want to have more frequent bowel movements, then you have to increase the amount of bulk (fiber) in your diet. Those words simply mean eating things that are not digestible and will increase the quantity of stool, and therefore the frequency of bowel movements. High-fiber diets are not difficult to follow. Many foods are prepared with extra fiber in them, and you can even add more in the form of bran. Once again, do not take a little and expect a miracle overnight. Eat those foods in quantity and give it some time. You can take stool softeners at the same time. A high-fiber diet seems to be especially important for the elderly who are prone to forming stools that are very pasty, so soft that the contractions of the bowel have little to push against. Almost all elderly patients of mine who have followed a truly high-fiber diet have found relief of their problem. It is a far better solution than laxatives.

Whatever your bowel complaint is, make it clear to your doctor. Be specific. You will not find much satisfaction if he does not understand the nature of your problem. Hard stools or infrequent bowel movements are usually not due to anything serious. *But any sudden unexplainable change in your bowel habits should be evaluated by a physician.*

Malignant tumors, carcinomas, of the large intestine are fairly common. Fortunately, they can be detected early, and are often curable by surgical removal in the early stages. There is more on the early diagnosis of this condition at the end of this chapter. Patients faced with the prospect of this kind of surgery are often concerned about the possibility of being left with a permanent colostomy, an opening in the abdomen through which the stool passes into a bag. Most of the time, that is not necessary. It is simply a question of where the tumor is. Most of the large intestine lies fairly free and loose in the abdomen. The very end and the rectum, however, are buried in the tissue of the pelvis. If the tumor is in a place where the involved section can be removed, leaving two ends that can be sewn together, then no colostomy is necessary. If it is near the rectum, however, the surgeon cannot just snip out a section, and a colostomy becomes necessary.

Let us turn our attention to the rest of the gastrointestinal tract, the liver, gall bladder, and pancreas.

The liver is a fairly large organ located in the right upper portion of the abdomen. Most of it is tucked up under the ribs. The liver receives the food absorbed from the small intestine, and, in simple terms, is an enormous and complex chemical factory. It also produces bile, which, as noted earlier, is necessary for the proper digestion of fats and oils.

Most diseases affecting the liver have to do with infection, alcohol, or malignancies. The most common infections are infectious hepatitis, which is caused by various viruses, and infectious mononucleosis, which is a much milder condition.

On a frequency basis, alcoholic liver disease may be the most common liver disorder of all. The basic facts are that excessive and continual alcoholic intake causes an ongoing and progressive inflammation of the liver that leads to cirrhosis. There is more on cirrhosis after the next paragraph.

Malignant tumors that begin in the liver are fairly uncommon, many of them beginning in livers that are already cirrhotic. The liver is, however, a place to which many different kinds of malignant tumors metastasize, or spread. Such a condition is, needless to say, ominous.

Cirrhosis of the liver simply means that the liver has become scarred either from an infection or chronic inflammation. Alcoholism and hepatitis are the two most common causes. If you want to understand the consequences of cirrhosis, you will have to know something about the blood circulation to the liver. It is a little complicated.

I mentioned earlier that the liver receives the absorbed food from the small intestine. How does it get there? Pay attention. Throughout most of the body, after blood has left the arterial system and perfused the tissues, it enters the venules. These join to form ever larger veins, which ultimately empty into the heart. Veins leaving the small intestine are an exception. The venules beginning in the small intestine form into what is called the portal vein. The portal vein enters the liver, and there begins to branch out again into microscopic vessels. This kind of circulation, beginning and ending with microscopic vessels, and not involving the heart, is called a portal circulation.

The scarring of cirrhosis impedes the flow of blood in this portal circulation, and raises the pressure in the portal vein system. Just as varicose veins form in the legs from an increase in venous blood pressure, so it happens in the portal system. The problem is that varicosities tend to form in the lower part of the esophagus, and have a tendency to bleed horrendously. Other problems that arise from an increase in pressure in the portal system are an enlargement of the spleen (the vein from the spleen goes into the portal vein), and a weeping of fluid into the abdominal cavity to form free-standing water, called ascites. That is the cause of the massively distended abdomens so commonly seen in patients with advanced liver disease. Needless to say, the problems that develop from advanced cirrhosis are many, difficult, and often ultimately fatal.

* * *

The gall bladder is a little sack under the liver, and is connected to it and the small intestine by ducts. Bile from the liver enters the gall bladder, is concentrated there, and is then released into the small intestine when we eat.

The common diseases of the gall bladder are stones and infections. The first thing to understand is that stones and infections go hand in hand. If you have one, you probably have the other, although neither may be serious enough to warrant doing anything about it. Stones become a problem when they either cause pain (colic) or move out into the bile duct and obstruct it. If either of these complications of having gall bladder stones persists, the gall bladder should be removed. Infection becomes a problem when it flares up and becomes acute. That also necessitates removal of the gall bladder.

Many patients are reluctant to have their gall bladder removed when advised to do so. They recite stories about friends having had theirs removed unnecessarily. That is sometimes the case, and I will have more to say about it. An infected gall bladder, however, is not a condition to play around with. Acute infection of the gall bladder can lead to its rupturing and infecting the entire abdominal cavity, or the infection can work its way into the liver, and that is very serious. This kind of decision that you may have to make one day is why it is important for you to have a personal physician you have confidence in. Remember, a lot of gall bladders are removed, and unnecessary surgery is the exception, not the rule.

Tests that can detect stones in the gall bladder include sonograms, CAT scans, and a test called a gall bladder series, which uses a contrast material that becomes concentrated in the gall bladder.

Now, what about gall bladders that are removed unnecessarily? If you are having upper abdominal problems, pains, discomforts, and are found to also have gall stones, that does not prove that the gall stones are causing your symptoms. Many a gall bladder has been removed for symptoms that later turn out to be due to an inflamed stomach or duodenum. It might be wise, depending, of course, on the nature and severity of your symptoms, to undergo a trial of therapy directed at gastritis and duodenitis first.

*   *   *

Before we go on to the pancreas, let us discuss jaundice. Jaundice is simply a yellowing of the skin due to elevated levels of a chemical called bilirubin in the blood. Bilirubin is the main element in bile, and is made in the spleen. It is an end product of the breakdown of hemoglobin from old red blood cells. Jaundice is not a disease. As with anemia and congestive heart failure, it is a condition that is always caused by an underlying disease.

There are three basic ways bilirubin can become increased in the blood. 1. There can be an obstruction to a bile duct and the bile backs up into the blood. 2. The liver can be so inflamed that it cannot remove from the blood the bilirubin coming to it from the spleen. 3. Red blood cells may die so fast (hemolytic anemia) that bilirubin is made faster than even a normal liver can remove it from the blood.

There is a simple way to know which of these processes is going on, especially the first and last. Bilirubin that has passed through the liver will dissolve in water, and if elevated in the blood, will appear in the urine, turning it very dark. This is called an obstructive jaundice. Bilirubin that has not passed through the liver, as in a hemolytic anemia, cannot get into the urine. This is called a hemolytic jaundice. There are, of course, many other tests that will make this kind of distinction. Inflammation of the liver, as in hepatitis, usually causes a mixture of both kinds of jaundice.

The pancreas is imbedded in the back wall of the upper abdomen, behind the lower stomach and duodenum. The bulk of the gland produces digestive enzymes that pass through a duct into the duodenum. There are "islets" of cells in the pancreas that produce insulin and other hormones related to sugar metabolism. These are secreted directly into the blood.

The two most common diseases of the pancreas are pancreatitis, a noninfectious inflammation, and malignant tumors of the pancreas. Pancreatitis can be a very painful and very serious illness. Most of the time it occurs in alcoholics and patients with gall bladder trouble. It is treated by putting the intestinal system, which includes the pancreas, completely at rest. Carcinomas of the pancreas are, unfortunately, among those malignancies that continue to defy early diagnosis and effective treatment.

Intestinal gas causes problems in many people, and symptoms caused by excessive amounts are many and varied. They include belching, sticking pains in the chest, sides, or back, cramps, and flatulence. Although there are serious conditions that can cause increased gas, such as gall bladder disease, ulcers, and diseases affecting the digestion of food, among others, the most common cause for excessive gas in my experience is air swallowing (aerophagia).

As I mentioned at the beginning of this chapter, we are supposed to swallow food that has been more or less liquefied in the mouth. If we swallow solid food, we also swallow the air that surrounds it. Reasons for swallowing excessive amounts of air include the lack of teeth, but far more commonly the lack of use of them, the hurried "two chomps and a swallow" meal. Pipe smoking and chewing gum can also cause this phenomenon. Once swallowed in quantity, air has to come out, one end or the other. Often, the air will cause distention of the intestines, and that can result in the sticking pains I mentioned above.

The most typical patient with this kind of problem is a male in his twenties or thirties who comes to the office complaining of sticking pains in his chest that he is certain are due to a heart attack. A few questions reveal that the pain is preceded by gulping his food, and often followed by a lot of noise from his rear.

In the absence of significant abdominal pain, abnormal bowel movements, or other associated symptoms, simple air swallowing is likely to be the culprit for your problem, so eat slowly and chew your food. The taking of simethicone during or immediately after a meal can help you belch the air up before it gets into your intestines.

The last topic for this chapter will be the subject of gastrointestinal bleeding, a not uncommon problem. There are many diseases that will cause bleeding within the G.I. tract. Most of these fall into the category of inflammatory diseases (including ulcers), diverticulitis, hemorrhoids, or malignancies. The manifestation of G.I. bleeding, in other words, what you see, depends upon where the bleeding is taking place, and how much blood is being lost.

Very active bleeding from the duodenum or above (upper G.I. bleeding) will result in the vomiting of red blood. If the blood lies in the stomach a while, it will turn dark and look like coffee grounds. The vomiting of blood is called hematemesis. The blood that passes through the intestines and comes out in the stool will turn the stool black, *if there is enough blood.* Passing a black stool due to blood is called melena.

Let us look at bleeding that originates below the duodenum. Bleeding from hemorrhoids is common and will result in fresh red blood that is usually seen in the toilet water and on the toilet paper. If you look closely, you will see that there is no blood mixed in the stool. Lower G.I. bleeding, meaning from the colon, can occasionally cause black stools, but more commonly dark or maroon blood mixed with the stool, *if there is enough blood.*

Pay attention to the following. *Any and all cases* of G.I. bleeding should be checked by a doctor. Remember, you can be bleeding significantly and continually and never see the blood in your stool. There has to be *a lot* of blood to turn the stool black! *There is no substitute for having your stool periodically chemically tested for blood.* In my practice, I average finding about one or two unsuspected cases of cancer of the colon a year simply by checking stools for blood, *and these cancers are often small and "curable"!*

Sometimes a patient will develop gastrointestinal bleeding, yet after every conceivable test is done, no definite site of the bleeding can be found. The degree of bleeding in these cases is usually minimal since there are tests that will detect the site of substantial bleeding. Also, this kind of problem is not usually due to a tumor, which would be readily findable. This condition of chronic G.I. bleeding can be very frustrating. Often the problem can be handled simply by treating the patient with injections of iron. If you will recall from the chapter on the blood, I mentioned that the bone marrow has the ability to produce more than a half pint's worth of red blood cells every day. Injections of iron may allow the patient to make blood fast enough to not become anemic from the bleeding.

CHAPTER 19

THE GENITOURINARY TRACT

The urinary tract consists of the kidneys; the ureters, which carry the urine from the kidneys to the bladder; the bladder itself; and the urethra, which conducts the urine from the bladder to the outside. We will also discuss a gland of the reproductive system, the prostate (*not* prostrate), and impotence.

The kidneys are buried in the back wall of the abdomen, in the flanks, a little above waist level. They serve to rid our bodies of toxic waste products. They are really remarkable organs, filtering an enormous amount of blood. Almost fifty gallons of water are removed from the blood in the kidneys every day. This is called the glomerular filtrate. Under normal circumstances, all of the valuable elements in this fluid (sugar for example), and almost all of the water, are reabsorbed into the blood. The small amount of water loaded with waste products that leaves the kidneys to be excreted is what we call urine.

There are many different diseases that can affect the kidneys. These include hypertension, diabetes, inflammatory diseases, infections, tumors, and obstructions to the outflow of urine, among others. We have three to four times more kidney tissue than we need to remain healthy, so any deterioration in kidney function will have no effect on us until the disease is quite advanced. Once that critical point is reached, however, things go rapidly downhill if the disease is progressive. Basically, the problems caused by poorly functioning kidneys are the same no matter which underlying disease caused the deterioration. The having of higher than normal levels of waste products in our blood is called azotemia. If the azotemia becomes severe enough to have some effect on our health, that is called chronic renal insufficiency. If that becomes worse, we enter into a state of uremia. We become poisoned by our own waste products. The common symptoms of uremia are fatigue, mental depression, loss of appetite and weight, and anemia. If the uremia becomes severe, it leads to death unless the patient is treated periodically with a dialysis machine, which removes the toxic waste products from the body. Routine blood tests done during a checkup include one or two tests that measure kidney function, a very good reason to have them done.

Once a patient is found to have a problem with kidney function, the underlying disease must be found. Sometimes it is obvious, such as untreated hypertension or diabetes. Other times the underlying disease is not obvious, and sometimes a needle biopsy of a kidney is necessary so a pathologist can discover which kidney disease is present.

The most common problems of the urinary tract result from infection, and obstruction to the flow of urine. Let us take a look at the various kinds of urinary tract infections, starting with the somewhat less serious (although not necessarily less uncomfortable).

The urethra is the tube that carries the urine from the bladder to the outside. In women it is very short. In men, however, it travels through the prostate and then through the entire length of the penis. Men, therefore, are subject to urethritis, an infection of the urethra. A woman who becomes infected with the same organism might get a vaginal or bladder infection. Symptoms of urethritis include a need to urinate often, a burning sensation when doing so, and often a penile discharge. Gonorrhea is the classic cause of urethritis. The acute symptoms of this infection usually go away even if untreated, but a minimal discharge will persist, usually in the mornings. Ultimately, the smouldering gonorrheal infection will cause scarring within the urethra that can lead to an obstruction to the voiding of urine. There are other microorganisms that commonly cause urethritis, but sometimes no organism is found.

I think it is important to emphasize here that it is not normal to experience *any* burning sensations when urinating. Often when I ask patients whether they have any such burning when they urinate, they will hesitate, then answer no. When I repeat the question, emphasizing the word *any*, they say, "Yes, but it's only occasional and slight." These patients invariably have some form of a mild urinary tract infection. (This is only one example of how patients frequently almost lie to a doctor. Can you understand a little better how important a careful history taking is?)

While we are on the subject of infections that are confined to men, we will discuss prostatitis, infection of the prostate. There will be more on the prostate and its diseases later in the chapter.

The prostate is situated at the base or outlet of the bladder. It functions as a prime contributor to seminal fluid. Much of the gland can be felt through the front wall of the rectum, a couple of inches up from the anus.

Prostatitis is a common problem, and most usually affects young men. It should not be confused with the condition that causes enlargement of the prostate, which often requires surgery in older men. Symptoms of prostatitis can include a mild burning sensation in the penis after urinating or ejaculating, or discomfort in the groin or perineal area (between the scrotum and anus). Occasionally men will experience discomfort when moving their bowels due to the stool in the rectum pressing on the gland. Sometimes the infection spreads to the bladder or towards the testes, infecting the tubules that transport sperm. Prostatitis is seldom a serious condition, although it does tend to be chronic and recurrent. Infrequent ejaculation is believed to be a major reason for the infection to develop. (Nature intended the human male to be very sexually active.) Treatment consists of antibiotics, heat, sometimes massage of the gland through the rectum, and frequent ejaculation.

Infections of the bladder (cystitis) occur in both sexes, but are far more common in women. That should not be surprising considering the great differences in the length of the urethra between the two sexes.

Cystitis in the female is not a cause for major concern if it is a single or very infrequent occurrence. If it occurs frequently, however, an evaluation by a urologist is definitely indicated. There may likely be an underlying problem predisposing the bladder to become infected. One of the more common reasons is urethral stenosis, which is discussed later. Many women, however, will suffer from repeated bouts of cystitis for no apparent reason, except possibly sex. Cystitis in brides is so common that it has been called "honeymoon cystitis." This problem is sometimes treated by taking a single dose of an antibiotic immediately after every sexual intercourse.

Cystitis in the male, even one occurrence, is a cause for concern, and requires a thorough investigation by a urologist for an underlying predisposing cause.

Acute pyelonephritis is an infection of a kidney, and is the most serious kind of urinary tract infection. In some cases, germs can escape into the blood and put the patient into shock. Here again, it is very important with even one episode of pyelonephritis that the urinary tract be checked for abnormalities that might predispose to getting an infection.

Chronic pyelonephritis, as might be guessed, is a chronic infection of a kidney. For some reason—usually a physical abnormality such as poor urine drainage or a stone sitting in the kidney—the kidney becomes infected again and again despite treatment with antibiotics. Chronic pyelonephritis can be treated with periodic administration of antibiotics for acute flare ups, continual administration of an antibiotic or a chemical that retards the growth of bacteria, or, in the most extreme case, surgical removal of the kidney, if, of course, the other kidney is healthy.

Let us turn to noninfectious problems of the urinary tract starting with the prostate.

The prostate gland causes more problems in men than the kidneys and bladder combined. As mentioned previously, it is located at the base or outlet of the bladder. There are three most common diseases of the prostate: infection, which we have discussed, malignant tumors, and benign enlargement.

Cancers of the prostate are much less common than benign enlargement. These tumors can often be detected early by a physician feeling the prostate through a rectal examination (another good reason for a periodic checkup!). Cancer of the prostate can often be cured by surgery, and even if it is incurable, it can often be well controlled for many, many years. Cancers of the prostate are often dependent upon the presence of male hormone to grow. Among the more common forms of treatment, therefore, is removal of the testes. This procedure eliminates the source of male hormone, and can arrest the growth of prostatic cancer that has spread. Female hormones are also often prescribed, and can put the cancer to rest. I have one patient whose bones have been riddled with cancer of the prostate for many years, but there has been little if any progression of the disease and he feels well. Removal of the testes and the taking of female hormones may not sound like a pleasant form of treatment, but most men with the condition are elderly, and it is a lot better than dying of the disease.

The very common prostate condition that causes difficulties with urinating in older men is called benign prostatic hypertrophy, often simply BPH. Simply stated, the gland slowly and progressively enlarges until it begins to block the outflow of urine from the bladder. The most common early symptom is frequent urination during the day and night. As the gland continues to enlarge, the force of the stream decreases, and the frequency of urination increases. The reason this happens is not difficult to understand. Although urine can be passed, the bladder cannot be emptied completely, therefore it simply fills up again more quickly. As the gland continues to enlarge there is often a delay, men having to wait a period of time until the urine begins to flow. In the extreme, an enlarged prostate can prevent the passing of urine competely.

I have to repeat something I mentioned elsewhere. Many patients do not understand the relationship and difference between the frequency of urination and the formation of urine. Patients of either sex who urinate frequently often look at me with confusion when I tell them that they need a water pill for some unrelated problem, stating: "But I urinate so frequently!" I am pleased about those who say this to me, because some keep quiet and simply never bother to take the water pill! Pay attention. As stated in the chapter on medications, water pills increase the amount of urine that is made in the kidneys and will be eliminated from the body. Problems with the prostate or bladder that cause you to urinate more frequently have nothing at all to do with the *amount* of urine being made.

The only treatment for BPH is surgery, which will be discussed a little later. (Sometimes, however, there is also a prostate infection present, and treatment of that will alleviate some of the obstructive symptoms.) The most important thing for you to understand is at what point surgery becomes a necessity. BPH is so common that one is tempted to say that it exists in all men past their fifties or sixties, but the simple presence of the condition is most definitely *not* an indication for surgery. Many men will find themselves getting up once or twice at night to urinate, maybe going to the bathroom one or two extra times during the day, or even perhaps having to wait a few seconds before the urine begins to flow. Problems of this degree do not warrant surgery because it is quite possible that the symptoms will not progress. Surgery does become necessary when complications arise, or, preferably, before that, when they "threaten" to arise. These complications include infection, complete obstruction, and physical damage to the bladder or kidneys.

A urinary tract infection is a common complication of an obstructing prostate. Since the bladder cannot be completely emptied, urine sort of stagnates there and becomes infected easily. Men will experience a burning sensation in the penis when urinating (dysuria). Treatment with antibiotics will usually eliminate the infection, but it is likely to come back, and soon. The development of a urinary tract infection in the presence of a significantly obstructing prostate is a definite indication for surgical relief of the obstruction. Failure to do so can result in very serious consequences. Infections may at first be confined to the bladder, but the inflammation resulting from the infection can further increase the obstruction, and ultimately the infection will progress upwards to the kidneys and infect one or both of those organs. When urine cannot drain properly from a kidney because of back pressure from an obstruction, the infection can get into the blood, and that can be a life-threatening situation.

Even if an infection does not develop, years of significant obstruction can result in permanent damage to the bladder and, of far greater importance, to the kidneys. When the symptoms progress to the point of having to urinate many times at night, or every hour during the day, or having the urine just dribble out, or having the urine come out on its own (incontinence), you have to get that obstruction relieved. You are soon likely to stop passing urine completely, and even if you do not, damage is being done, and much of it may be irreversible. At the very least, delaying treatment of these kinds of problems will result in markedly prolonged hospital stays.

The most common surgery for an obstructing prostate is done through the penis. This is called a transurethral resection of the prostate, a TURP. Sometimes, because of the size of the gland or other urological considerations, the gland must be removed by a somewhat more complicated surgical procedure. A suprapubic, or the similar retropubic, prostatectomy is done through an incision in the lower abdomen just above the pubic bone.

The subject of prostate surgery usually raises the question of possible sexual complications. It is true that retrograde ejaculation is a common consequence. That means that the seminal fluid goes into the bladder instead of coming out through the penis. This will result in sterility but not impotence. Whether true impotence can result from prostate surgery is a somewhat controversial question because some men claim to have that side effect. The medical consensus, and my opinion, is that it does not.

Urethral stenosis is, in a sense, the female counterpart of an obstructing prostate. It is very common, but a less serious condition. It is simply a partial closure or blockage of the urethra, usually due to chronic inflammation and scarring. Symptoms are very similar to an obstructing prostate in men, including frequent urination, dribbling of the urinary stream, and recurrent infection.

The treatment for urethral stenosis is usually nothing more than a simply and relatively painless dilation procedure done in a urologist's office. The condition, however, is *usually recurrent*, and women with this problem should have it checked by a urologist once or twice a year. If left untreated, there is the potential for bladder damage and infection spreading up to the kidneys. A few years ago a patient of mine with recurrent bladder infections and symptoms of urethral stenosis ignored my advice to see a urologist. Two weeks later she developed shaking chills, a temperature of 104 degrees, and quickly went into shock from bacteria escaping into her blood from an infected kidney. A trip to the urologist's office would have been a lot easier than her two weeks in the hospital.

Kidney stones are a very common, and very painful, affliction. But that is not quite true. Although stones form in the kidney, they do not usually cause pain until they begin to pass, until they get into the ureter, which, as noted, is the tube connecting the kidney to the bladder. There are two most common kinds of kidney stones, calcium and uric acid, and there is a marked difference between what is necessary to find them, what other tests have to be done, and sometimes in their treatment.

Calcium stones are often visible on a plain X-ray, just as the calcium in bones is. Uric acid stones cannot be seen on a plain X-ray. An intravenous pyelogram is a series of kidney X-rays done after the injection of a contrast material into the blood. This material is excreted by the kidneys and makes them, the ureters, and the bladder visible. A uric acid stone will show up as a dark spot in an opaque ureter.

If a patient has a tendency to form calcium stones, his serum calcium level should be checked, and a condition called hyperparathyroidism, which predisposes to the formation of calcium stones, should be looked for (see Chapter 21). If a patient has a uric acid stone, his serum uric acid level should be checked, and quite possibly he should be treated with allopurinol, as described in the section on gout in Chapter 12.

Finally, calcium is more soluble in acid urine, so patients with calcium stones need to eat and drink things that make their urine more acid. Uric acid is more soluble in alkaline urine, so obviously you do not want to go out of your way to acidify your urine if you have that type of stone.

Whatever the stone is made of, it hurts the same. The pain from a stone passing through a ureter is among the most intense pains known. It can run from the flank in the back where the kidney is, around and down to the groin and testes. There is a general tendency for the pain to follow the stone. If most of your pain is in the back, the stone is still near the kidney. If you are feeling most of the pain in the front and groin, the stone is probably near the bladder, and once it pops into it, the pain will disappear. The stone will usually be passed from the bladder with little difficulty.

The treatment for a passing kidney stone consists of drinking enough fluids to almost drown yourself in an attempt to flush out the stone, and time. Most kidney stones will pass by themselves, but it might take a few days. Surgical or endoscopic intervention by a urologist is only necessary if the stone becomes stuck.

Physical sexual problems occur in both sexes. In females this problem is most commonly painful intercourse (dyspareunia). One common cause is dry vaginal tissues in postmenopausal women. This condition can be alleviated by the judicious use of female hormonal (estrogen) creams, a safe form of treatment in most women. If this is not the cause, an evaluation by a gynecologist is indicated because many other conditions can result in painful intercourse, such as infections of the Fallopian tubes (salpingitis) or ovarian problems.

Sexual dysfunction in the male is usually the inability to develop an erection (impotence). Causes of this condition include the side effects of certain medications, diabetes, arterial problems, hormonal problems, and, most commonly, psychologic factors. If the underlying cause of the impotence cannot be treated or helped, the choice boils down to either forgoing sexual intercourse or having a penile implant.

There are basically two types of penile implants. The simplest procedure consists of the implanting of plastic rods in the penis. Contrary to what many men seem to imagine, the result is not a rigid, stiff, and protruding organ, but rather a penis only firm enough to allow vaginal penetration. The penis does not stand fully out but rather folds down relatively inconspicuously.

The more complicated types of penile prostheses allow an erection on demand. I have had minimal professional experience with these. It is my understanding that the older kinds required much more extensive surgery. A fluid reservoir had to be implanted in the lower abdomen. The more modern variety consists of a self-contained system entirely within the penis, and is preferred by the urologist I have spoken with.

It is something of a mystery to me why more impotent men do not have this done. Often, when I discuss the subject with patients, I see an initial positive response followed by a statement of procrastination. Perhaps they are embarrassed. Several of my patients have had a penile implant, and all have been thoroughly satisfied.

CHAPTER 20

INFECTION

An infection means that a foreign microorganism, a germ of some kind, has invaded your body. Fortunately, your body itself will kill and eliminate these organisms almost all the time.

There are a wide variety of different classes and kinds of microorganisms that can be infectious. These include viruses, bacteria, and yeasts and molds, among many, many others. Most microorganisms in the world cannot cause infections. Some can only do so when a person is vulnerable for one reason or another, such as with a poorly functioning immune system, a low white-blood-cell count, or alcoholism. Others cause infection frequently, but are readily and rapidly destroyed by the body's natural defenses. Cold viruses are an example of this. Some microorganisms are virulent and can cause permanent injury or death.

What are the body's natural defenses against infection? The first would have to be exclusion. Our skin and mucous membranes serve as a barrier to organisms entering our body. There are also protective measures at the openings and in the passages into our bodies. The tonsils in the throat, and tissues just inside the anus, are rich in lymphocytes, a type of white blood cell. Mucus is secreted in the trachea and bronchi, and is always being propelled out of the body by microscopic hairlike "cilia." Tears and semen contain chemicals that can kill microorganisms. Our bodies even use harmless microorganisms to protect us from ones that can cause disease. The vagina is normally loaded with a bacterium called lactobacillus, the presence of which inhibits the growth of other microorganisms. The same thing holds true for the large intestine, a whole host of "normal" bacteria helping to suppress the growth of those that may be harmful.

Once a microorganism does invade our body, our white blood cells spring into action. As mentioned in an earlier chapter, some actually eat and digest foreign organisms. Others begin the process of producing antibodies, protein chemicals that stick to the microorganism and either kill it or render it more susceptible to being eaten.

"Localization and confinement" is another body defense. If we cut ourselves and get an infection, the body immediately begins to try to wall off the infected area, to isolate it from the rest of the body, and ultimately to work the entire area to the surface and expel it. An abscess that ultimately breaks open is a classic example of this. If the infection does begin to spread, the nearest lymph glands, such as those in the armpit or groin, come into play, again acting as a wall against further spread. This process even takes place inside the abdomen. The loose membranes that support the intestine, the mesentery, can be very effective in surrounding, walling off, and isolating an area of infection. Perhaps the classic example of wall building is with tuberculosis in the lungs. Classically, when a tuberculosis germ begins an infection, the body reacts by forming a fibrous barrier around it, which then becomes calcified, a "cement" wall visible on an X-ray as a tubercle.

If our natural defense mechanisms against infections are inadequate, we have to turn to the artificial. We enjoy today the ability to make ourselves immune with vaccinations to many of the more virulent kinds of microorganisms. Others we know how to protect ourselves against by disposing of sewage properly and keeping disease-carrying insects and animals away from us. Certainly the long life span we enjoy today as compared to centuries ago is due primarily to our ability to protect ourselves from infections, and cure most of those we get.

Our weapons of last resort against microorganisms invading our bodies are antibiotics. Some microorganisms, viruses for example, are unaffected by antibiotics, a good reason why these medications will not help the common cold or the flu. Most other organisms that cause infection, however, are controlled by antibiotics, so let us discuss the common misconceptions about those weapons. They were discussed in Chapter 8, but they could bear repeating.

The first thing to understand is that *there is no antibiotic that will cure an infection by itself. The active participation of the body's natural defenses is an absolute necessity.* It would be wonderful to have a pill that immediately killed every bad germ in our body, but such a thing does not exist.

Another popular misconception about antibiotics is evidenced by the frequently stated: "That antibiotic doesn't work on me," or "I'm immune to antibiotics." Antibiotics have nothing to do with *you*, unless you are allergic to one, or it upsets your stomach. The antibiotic is for the microorganism, and it is that little fellow it may or may not work on. If you had the experience of an antibiotic not working, it is likely your infection was caused by a virus. It is true, however, that many microorganisms are resistant to one kind of antibiotic or another. There is more on this a little later. We learn which antibiotics kill which germs by culturing as described in Chapter 7. Fortunately, we have many antibiotics to choose from. Some, however, can only be administered by injection because there is no pill form.

Another frequent point of confusion among patients is that they think they are taking an antibiotic for a fever. That is not the case. Antibiotics have no direct effect on fever. They only reduce fever by helping to get rid of the infection, *and antibiotics can often take as long as several days to have their full effect!*

Let us talk a little more about fever. The body temperature is regulated by a part of the brain. When it detects a pyrogen (fever producer) in the blood, it raises our temperature and gives us fever. Pyrogens are chemical by-products of an infection or inflammation. The reason fever exists is probably to increase our general metabolism. Our cells work faster if slightly hotter, and may allow us to fight off the invading germ more quickly. Another possible reason for fever is that germs probably grow best at our normal body temperature, and a hotter body may make them less active. There are circumstances where the body temperature will not rise in response to an infection. This sometimes happens in the very elderly, and also in anyone when the infection is overwhelming. In the former, the absence of fever obviously makes the infection difficult to diagnose. In the latter, the absence of fever is a very ominous sign.

Many times I will ask patients with symptoms of an infection if they have had fever, and they answer no. Maybe they have even taken their temperature and found it to be normal. Then I will ask them if they have had any chills or sweats, and they answer yes. Understand that if you have had chills followed by sweats, you have had at least some fever in between. You just did not take your temperature at the right time. Many people seem to think that fever is a steady-state condition, but that's an uncommon situation. Most of the time when we are infected, our body temperature rises and falls periodically during the day. We feel chilly, or in the extreme get a chill that makes us shake, then our temperature rises above normal, then we sweat, and the temperature drops, sometimes down to normal. Some time later, the cycle begins again.

It has been my experience that many people pay too much attention to fever, as if the fever itself is the primary problem rather than just the result of an infection. Their thoughts and energies are confined to bringing the fever down, by any means, as if that by itself would mean that their infection is cured. Fever is only the by-product of an infection, and driving it down, as with the use of aspirin, may make you feel better, but it does nothing to the infection itself.

While we're on the subject of fever, what is a normal body temperature? How high does it have to go to be called "fever"? How much of a difference is there between oral and rectal temperature? To answer the last question first. Rectal temperatures are about half a degree warmer than oral. Normal body temperature taken orally is anywhere from about 98 degrees, or even a little lower, up to 99.5 degrees. I consider any temperature between 99.5 degrees and 100.5 degrees to be low-grade fever, although it is probable that some people could have a normal body temperature up to 100 degrees.

Those common infections that we do get are usually caused by only one, or a few, different kinds of germs. That is why your doctor usually knows if an antibiotic will help, and which ones to prescribe. This situation often changes when an infection becomes chronic. A different germ may take over as the primary infecting organism, and it quite likely will be resistant to the antibiotics that worked before. An example of this would be urinary tract infections. The germ causing a first bladder infection in a healthy woman would almost always be sensitive to many different commonly used antibiotics. If that woman develops a chronic kidney infection over the years, the germs will change, and may only be sensitive to seldom-used antibiotics that must be given by injection.

It is your doctor's decision as to whether you should take an antibiotic or not. I am not in favor of patients deciding on their own to take an antibiotic.

Let us take a look at some of the more common infections that have not been discussed elsewhere in this book.

Upper respiratory infections (colds) are certainly the most common form of infection. They are caused by viruses, and cannot be helped by an antibiotic. It should be remembered, however, that a bacterial infection of the lungs, or sinuses, or ear, can follow on the heels of a cold virus, and they should be treated with an antibiotic.

The treatment of a common cold is symptomatic. Take aspirin or acetaminophen, decongestants and cough medicine if necessary, and wait for it to go away.

One note of caution. If you have a severe sore throat, and are assuming it is due to a cold, you might be overlooking a strep throat. Streptococcus is a bacterial cause of a sore throat, and is important not because of the throat infection, but because of the possible complications of either rheumatic fever, which can damage the heart valves, or acute glomerulonephritis, which can damage the kidneys. If your throat is bad, see your doctor. He may do a throat culture to determine if streptococcus is present. With or without a culture, treatment with penicillin or other antibiotics will eradicate strep if it is there.

Gastrointestinal viral infections are very common. The stomach or the intestines or both may be involved. Symptoms can include any or all of the following: fever, nausea, vomiting, cramps, and diarrhea. These infections can last a day or a week. Remember, there are other kinds of germs that can cause intestinal infections, especially in infants and in foreign lands. If you are not too sick, it is fine to wait a few days to see if it is going to go away. If you are very ill, see your doctor. I recently had an unhappy experience with an elderly woman. She had been experiencing diarrhea for weeks at home, refusing to see a doctor. By the time her family brought her to the emergency room, she was so far gone from dehydration that she quickly died. Had we had a day or so to treat her, it is quite likely she might have survived. Antispasmodics are commonly prescribed for these types of viral illnesses.

The flu is also caused by viruses, and like cold viruses, they change from year to year. That is why new flu vaccines are formulated every year. It is not necessary for most people to take those shots, unless there is a particularly virulent virus coming our way. The elderly, however, along with diabetics, patients with chronic lung disease, and others who are more susceptible to the complications of the flu, such as pneumonia, should have flu shots yearly.

Shingles is a viral infection about which many patients are confused. It is caused by the virus that causes chicken pox, and it develops in patients who have had the disease but who are only partially immune. In shingles, the virus infects the nerves. It is not uncommon for pain or burning to be felt in the area of the infection for a few days before anything becomes visible on the skin. The virus follows along the path of the nerve, raising tiny clear blisters as it does. These blisters eventually break, leaving the skin raw until it heals over. The classic appearance of shingles is a line of blisters and raw areas on one side of the body only. Unfortunately, I know of no effective treatment for this infection. You just have to wait for it to go away.

Boils, medically called furuncles, are the curse of many people. These red and swollen skin abscesses are a nuisance, and are painful. A boil begins when a sebaceous cyst becomes infected. A sebaceous cyst forms when the duct of one of the innumerable microscopic oil glands in the skin becomes clogged. The lining of the gland continues to secrete oil, and the result is a progressively enlarging cyst filled with dried oil. When staphylococcus, a normal skin bacterium, gets inside it finds an excellent material in which to grow. Opening and draining the boil, along with heat and antibiotics, is the usual treatment. If the infection recurs, the entire cyst should be surgically removed. If you are prone to this problem, try to keep those areas of your skin clean with something rough and abrasive, and use an antibacterial soap. It may help.

Cellulitis is an infection of the skin. It most commonly occurs in the lower legs in patients who have edema, broad areas becoming red, swollen, and painful. Unlike a boil, where the infection is localized and isolated by the body, the germs causing cellulitis contain enzymes that break down the body's barrier and allow the infection to spread. Cellulitis can cause a high fever and requires intensive medical care.

Although internal infections with fungi are uncommon, the skin is very susceptible. In case you do not understand what a fungus is, it is the same kind of organism as a mold, the stuff you see growing on food kept around the house too long. The skin infections I am referring to here are athlete's foot, ringworm, and those rashes we humans get in the groin, the armpits, under the breasts, and under hanging fat in the excessively obese. A fungus can only grow where it is damp, hence the predilection for the above areas. Natural treatment includes keeping the area dry and exposing it to the sun. There are also many different kinds of creams and ointments, prescription and nonprescription, that contain fungicides—medication that will kill the fungus. Under extreme conditions, there is a medication taken in pill form that gets into the skin and kills the fungus very effectively.

The space under the toenails is particularly susceptible to fungus growth, and it is difficult for creams or ointments to penetrate very deeply. Very often the best bet is to remove the dead area of the nail to expose the space beneath to the air. The oral medication I mentioned before is very effective in eliminating fungus under the toenails, but it has to be taken for many months, and once stopped, the fungus may simply begin to grow again.

The space under the fingernails used to be a very rare place to get a fungus infection since it is exposed to the air and usually dry. More and more women, however, are gluing artificial nails to their natural ones, and prolonged use of them seems to markedly predispose to fungal infection. If that is happening to you, you had better stop using artificial nails now. You are going to have to stop eventually, because the fungal infection is only going to get worse, and your fingers are going to start to hurt.

The vagina is susceptible to two common kinds of infections. Moniliasis, or candidiasis, is a yeast that can grow in the vagina. It causes a discharge of thick white "cheesy" material. The most common conditions that predispose to getting this kind of infection are poorly controlled diabetes, and the taking of an antibiotic that kills off the lactobacillus I mentioned earlier. The insertion of suppositories or creams containing a fungicide eliminates the infection.

Trichomonas is another common cause of vaginal infection. This microorganism is actually a one-celled animal with a whiplike tail that propels it around. Many women have the organism in their vaginas without it causing much in the way of symptoms other than a slight watery vaginal discharge. More severe infections bring on vaginal burning. This infection is treated with a pill that kills the microorganism, but a word of caution. The organism can easily live in the sex glands of men, where it rarely causes any symptoms. It is wise for women who have the infection to make certain that their bed partner takes the medication at the same time they do.

CHAPTER 21

DIABETES AND THE ENDOCRINE SYSTEM

The endocrine system is a group of widely separated, but inter-related, glands that secrete hormones into the blood. These glands include the pituitary, the thyroid, the parathyroids, the adrenals, the pancreas, the ovaries, and the testes. These glands regulate much of our metabolism (our chemical processes), as well as our reproductive ability, and urges. Needless to say, they are extremely important!

We are going to devote the bulk of our discussion to the two most common kinds of disorders within this system, diabetes, including a brief discussion of hypoglycemia, and problems with the thyroid, but first a very brief overall view.

The pituitary gland sits under the brain. It has historically been called the master gland because it controls other endocrine glands. The pituitary itself is controlled by a part of the brain. Many of the different hormones the pituitary secretes force other glands to work harder, to do their thing, so to speak. The pituitary also plays a central role in the complex hormonal mechanisms that lead to growth, ovulation, menstruation, pregnancy, milk formation in the breasts, and male potency.

There are four parathyroid glands, each imbedded in a corner of the thyroid gland in the neck. They are the prime regulators of the amount of calcium in the blood. The dietary intake of calcium has essentially no effect on this. Calcium is a very important and very active element. Seemingly minor increases or decreases in the blood can wreak havoc.

Too much parathyroid hormone (hyperparathyroidism) increases the blood calcium and causes a multitude of problems including mental confusion, ulcers, bone wasting, and stone formation in the kidneys. This condition is often found by accident, when routine blood tests reveal an elevated calcium level, and is a good argument for having periodic checkups. Too little parathyroid hormone (hypoparathyroidism) is much less common. This causes a decrease in the blood calcium and causes severe muscle spasms, among other problems. (I am not talking about nighttime muscle cramps in the legs!)

There is one adrenal gland sitting on top of each kidney. Each adrenal is really two glands in one. The center secretes adrenaline and other similar hormones. The outer layers are controlled by the pituitary and secrete cortisone (yes, cortisone is a natural hormone, and is necessary for life!) and other hormones related to it.

The ovaries and testes secrete female and male sex hormones respectively, and work in an interrelationship with the pituitary.

I am not going to delve into the subject of diabetes in great depth. I just want to provide a general understanding of the disease and its treatment, and to clear up a few prevalent misconceptions.

What is diabetes? The word *diabetes* actually means a "passing through," in other words, quickly urinating out fluids that have been taken in. This is an example of a disease named by physicians of a far earlier age. The disease we are talking about specifically is diabetes mellitus, "sweet" diabetes. There is a condition called diabetes insipidus which has nothing to do with sugar at all.

The kind of diabetes mellitus that strikes children (juvenile diabetes) is quite different from the condition we see developing in older adults as they age (adult onset diabetes). In the former, there is an absolute lack of insulin secretion by the pancreas. In the latter, insulin is secreted, but does not work normally.

Sugar, more specifically the sugar glucose (there are many different kinds of sugars) is literally our fuel of life. Our cells burn glucose in a controlled stepwise manner to get heat and energy.

Many people find it hard to understand how their blood sugar can be too high if they do not eat sugar. The explanation is not very complicated. One way we can get sugar is to manufacture it inside our bodies. We have the chemical ability to convert proteins into sugar, and this can become a substantial process if we are deprived of dietary sugar. The major way we get sugar is in the form of starch. Starch, such as in rice, bread, and potatoes, is nothing more than a connected series of sugar molecules. If sugar were a bead, starch would be a bead necklace. Enzymes in our intestines break the string, so to speak. They digest starch into individual molecules of sugar.

We absorb glucose into the blood from the small intestine, but it does not pass easily from the blood to the insides of our cells. That is where insulin comes into play. Insulin is secreted into the blood by the pancreas, and markedly increases the movement of glucose into cells. Under normal conditions, the pancreas senses how much glucose is in our blood, and secretes the appropriate amount of insulin. When there is not enough insulin, glucose cannot get into the cells, and it accumulates in the blood.

What are normal blood sugar levels? I will not be very specific to save myself the wrath of diabetologists and laboratory directors. If you have not eaten for several hours, your "fasting" blood sugar should be in the range of 60 to 115, and even if you have eaten candy and ice cream constantly for hours, it should not be higher than about 160.

Does the *absence* of sugar in the urine prove that there is no diabetes?' Absolutely not, although the *presence* of sugar in your urine quite likely means that you do have diabetes. If you will recall from the chapter on the kidneys, I mentioned that they absorb sugar in the urine back into the blood. In most people, the kidneys can reabsorb all urine sugar unless the blood sugar is well over 200. Only then will sugar appear in the urine. Since a blood sugar above 160 is not normal, you can easily have diabetes without having sugar in the urine.

Does the presence of a normal fasting blood sugar prove the absolute absence of diabetes? Not really. The absence of diabetes can only be shown conclusively by demonstrating normal glucose tolerance, and that kind of testing becomes complicated. Most physicians, however, including myself, settle for a routine normal fasting blood sugar as showing the absence of diabetes.

What is a diabetic? Many of my patients, when I tell them that their blood sugar is higher than normal, will say: "But that doesn't mean I have diabetes, does it?" The definition of diabetes is a matter of some controversy. I like the concept that anyone who has shown, or will show, an inability to normally metabolize sugar is a diabetic. That philosophy can go as far as saying that if both of your parents have or had diabetes, you are a diabetic, no matter what your current blood sugars are. This is only applying a label to someone, not giving him a disease. The other side of the semantic coin is the term "glucose or carbohydrate intolerance." This is used by some physicians to describe patients who have a minimal abnormality of sugar metabolism, and who are not prone to the long-term complications of diabetes.

The symptoms of diabetes are related to the metabolic problem, glucose not getting into the cells properly, accumulating in the blood, and passing into the urine. A lack of enough glucose to burn causes weakness and fatigue, and also hunger. As far as the body is concerned, it is starving! Glucose in the urine acts as a diuretic. It pulls water out of the body, creating frequent or constant thirst. This sugar that is lost in the urine represents food that has been eaten, but not used, so weight loss is common. Under more extreme conditions, when essentially no glucose is entering the cells, the body has to rely on burning fat exclusively for heat and energy. The burning of fat is a normal ongoing process in everyone, but when fat is burned to excess, the by-products, acetone and acids, accumulate. That leads to the condition called diabetic ketosis or to diabetic ketoacidosis. The latter condition, when severe, can be fatal.

The word *brittle* is used to describe some diabetics. A brittle diabetic is one who can pass very easily and quickly into a state of ketosis or ketoacidosis, and then conversely into a state of having an excessively low blood sugar. This is a difficult problem to take care of, and usually happens only in those affected with the juvenile form of diabetes.

Other symptoms of diabetes are related to long-term complications, the effects of diabetes on the eyes, the kidneys, the arteries, and the nerves. Most are discussed or mentioned elsewhere in this book, in the chapters relating to those organs.

Once you have diabetes, you should be treated for it in some manner.

There are four basic kinds of therapy for diabetes: diet, weight loss, pills, and insulin. Diet is essential no matter the state of your diabetes. Sometimes it is the only treatment necessary. The essence of it is that you should keep your sugar intake minimal and your carbohydrate, or starch, intake reasonable.

If you are overweight, then calorie control comes into the picture. Excess body fat markedly increases the need for insulin, among the many other adverse effects it has. Do not allow the brevity of this statement to mislead you into thinking that getting rid of excess fat is not very important. It is!

Diabetics who have had glycosuria (sugar in the urine), and are then brought under control with medication, have a particularly rough time when it comes to weight. They have been eating enormous quantities of food to compensate for what they have been losing in the urine. Once they no longer have glycosuria, their food requirement becomes a very small fraction of what they are used to eating. Rapid weight gain, unfortunately, is not an uncommon complication of the treatment of diabetes!

When diabetes cannot be controlled by diet and weight loss, medication becomes necessary. In most, but not all, adult onset diabetics, pills are used, at least at the beginning. All antidiabetic pills do the same thing. They initially stimulate the pancreas to produce more insulin, and then have an effect on the liver to decrease the production of glucose. (There is no pill form of insulin. It must be given by injection, although new delivery systems are on the horizon.) Their effectiveness is limited by the ability of the pancreas to respond. Antidiabetic pills have little or no effect in juvenile diabetes. In adult onset diabetes, they may work well initially, but then become less and less effective as time passes. It is the nature of adult onset diabetes that blood sugars tend to rise as you get older, so get rid of that fat!

Insulin becomes necessary when the pills are no longer effective in maintaining an acceptable blood sugar. Notice, I said "acceptable," not normal. Running the risk of assassination by the diabetologists again, I consider a fasting blood sugar of 150 or less to be acceptable.

There are many differing opinions on how insulin should be given.

These range from a once-a-day administration of a long-acting insulin, to twice a day, to multiple injections of a short-acting insulin. It would seem logical that the best theoretical way to administer insulin would be several times a day, whenever food is eaten. After all, that would be the best imitation of what happens naturally. Such regimens are often necessary in the juvenile brittle diabetic and the pregnant diabetic. Whether it makes for a significantly healthier patient with insulin-dependent adult onset diabetes, whether it will prevent or delay the onset of the later complications of diabetes such as eye, kidney, and vascular problems, is controversial. Until it is shown that that is the case, I do not see that the disease is better controlled, in most patients, by more than one administration of insulin a day, at least not to the point where it is worth the time, effort, and extra needles.

I cannot recall one patient of mine who liked the idea of switching from pills to insulin. It is certainly understandable. No one likes needles. Let me hasten to add, however, that after patients do make that switch, they rarely want to go back to pills because they feel so much better, even if they have not felt that bad to begin with! I remember a woman I saw in consultation. She had been admitted to the hospital with a urinary tract infection by a urologist who called me in to take care of her diabetes, which was very poorly controlled by diabetic pills. I told her she had to be treated with insulin, permanently. She did not like the idea, but reluctantly accepted it. When I told her that she was going to feel a lot better, however, she looked at me as if I were crazy, stating that, aside from her burning when she urinated, she felt fine, that she could not possibly feel any better. Three or four days later, she greeted me with a large smile of wonder and amazement, stating that she could not believe how much stronger she felt! The basic fact of life is that insulin is better for you than the pills. Diabetics well controlled on insulin are healthier than those on oral medications. So if your doctor tells you that he thinks you would do better on insulin, do not argue with him.

Control of your food intake is especially important when you are taking insulin. Once you have injected insulin into yourself, especially a long-acting form that will function in your body for a full twenty-four hours or longer, you must eat at fairly frequent intervals or else your blood sugar may fall too low. Feeling weak and sweaty, perhaps with a headache, can lead to passing out and even convulsions. I repeatedly warn my patients taking insulin as to the necessity of eating at regular intervals, as often as six times a day, and of the symptoms of this hypoglycemia. I insist that they always have sugar pills with them at all times, just in case.

Diabetics should test their urine for sugar periodically, if their blood sugars show a tendency to go high enough to cause glycosuria. The past years have seen more and more diabetics testing their own blood sugars at home to regulate their insulin dosage. For the patients I care for, I do not see that it adds that much to the management of the disease, again, at least not enough to warrant all those finger sticks. It is, however, an important aid to the management of a brittle diabetic.

In discussing the treatment of diabetes, I mentioned the opposite condition, hypoglycemia, low blood sugar. I have also mentioned hypoglycemia in the nondiabetic in an earlier chapter. It was quite a fashionable diagnosis at one time, and, I believe, diagnosed far in excess of its actual prevalence. There are basically two kinds of hypoglycemia, fasting and reactive. In the first kind, the blood sugar drops too low after a prolonged period of not eating. I have had only one documented case in eighteen years of practice. The second kind is supposed to be more common. The sugar drops too low several hours after eating because of an oversecretion of insulin. It is supposed to be worse when sugar is eaten and may be the first sign of diabetes. I have checked any number of patients for this condition, including many who had previously been told that they had it, but I have actually found it in very few. The condition certainly exists, but in my humble opinion there are a lot of doctors who have been making this diagnosis when it is not warranted.

The thyroid gland is located in the front of the neck, just above the little V between your collar bones, and below your Adam's apple. It produces a hormone called, naturally, thyroid hormone. There are really two closely related thyroid hormones called T3 and T4. Enough about that. Thyroid hormone is one of the prime regulators of our metabolism; too much turns it up, too little turns it down. The thyroid gland produces thyroid hormone on command from the master gland, the pituitary. When the pituitary senses that there is not enough thyroid hormone in the blood, it produces more "thyroid stimulating hormone" (TSH). If there is too much thyroid hormone in the blood, the pituitary stops secreting TSH.

Even those patients with a degree of medical sophistication seem to be inevitably confused when trying to understand the relationship between the *activity* of the thyroid (the production of thyroid hormone) and its *size*. The reason is simple. There is none.

The most common thyroid problems fall into two basic categories, the size of the gland, and the function of the gland. The thyroid can be normal sized, diffusely enlarged, or have a nodule or nodules. It can be normally active, overactive, or underactive. To repeat, there is no consistent connection between the size of the thyroid gland and its function or activity. Any size gland can be normally active, or overactive or underactive, depending upon the particular disorder.

When a thyroid is producing too much hormone the condition is called hyperthyroidism. The excess hormone may be produced by a gland that is only minimally enlarged, greatly enlarged, or by one that merely has a small overactive nodule. Most of the symptoms are the same. They usually consist of losing weight while you are eating ravenously, feeling hot and sweating when others around you are cool, palpitations, a fine trembling in your hands, and, in the case of women, scanty menstrual periods. I had one patient a few years ago, a young man, whose only symptom of hyperthyroidism was severe weakness in his thigh muscles. The classic kind of hyperthyroidism is called Grave's disease, and is associated with a bulging of the eyes.

The treatment for an overactive gland usually consists of either drugs that can reduce the production of the hormones, or a single dose of radioactive iodine that destroys much of the gland over a period of time. Sometimes surgery is necessary. I prefer the radioactive-iodine form of treatment when possible, unless the patient is a woman who is likely to become pregnant. It is simpler and safer than the drugs, even though it usually leads to the thyroid becoming underactive. More on that below. The drugs for an overactive gland have a potential to be toxic, and frequent blood tests are necessary to check on them.

When a thyroid gland is producing too little hormone the condition is called hypothyroidism. Such a problem can be caused by the failure of the pituitary to produce its thyroid-stimulating hormone, but usually the problem is with the thyroid itself, and TSH levels in the blood are very high as the pituitary tries to whip a failing gland. Again, in hypothyroidism the thyroid may be markedly enlarged or basically normal in size. Common symptoms include sluggishness, weight gain, puffiness of the face, and heavy menstrual periods. This disorder, in its milder form, is often unsuspected, first detected through routine blood tests.

Many overweight patients express a belief that they must have a hormonal disorder to account for their inability to lose weight, that their thyroid must be giving them a sluggish metabolism. There is nothing wrong with having thyroid blood tests—I do them routinely—but do not expect them to be abnormal. It is almost always a case of wishful thinking on the part of an overeater.

The treatment of an underactive gland is very simple. You just take thyroid hormone in pill form. The amount you need is easily determined by blood tests, and once the right dose has been established you can basically forget about it, as long as you take the pills. Sometimes new patients will tell me that they see a thyroid specialist once every month or two for this condition. Unlike the frequent checks that are necessary when taking medication for an overactive thyroid, that is completely unnecessary for an underactive gland. A once-a-year check on your thyroid is more than sufficient.

Now let us look at the thyroid gland from a viewpoint of its size. If a diffusely enlarged gland is so big that it makes your neck bulge (a goiter), you want it shrunk. If it is underactive, or even normally active, the taking of thyroid hormone in pill form will usually make it shrink and is completely safe. If the gland is overactive, radioactive iodine will probably make it shrink. Sometimes surgery is necessary. If, however, the problem is that you have a nodule in your thyroid, there is now the possibility of having a tumor. The likelihood of it being a tumor or not can often be determined by tests, but sometime the best and safest thing to do is have the nodule removed.

There are other kinds of thyroid problems such as benign and malignant tumors, and inflammatory diseases, but they are relatively uncommon.

CHAPTER 22

PSYCHOSOMATIC DISORDERS

I have asked many of my patients if they understood what I mean when I say that a condition is psychosomatic, or that it is emotional, or due to anxiety or tension. Usually I do that when I see them become annoyed or defensive when I use those words. I cannot recall one who really understood what psychosomatic means. Some expressed their belief that I was telling them they were crazy. Others had the impression that I was telling them that their complaints were all in their imagination. Still others thought I was accusing them of faking. Well, neither insanity, imagination, nor fakery has anything to do with psychosomatic disorders. "Psycho" refers to the mind. "Soma" refers to the body. Psychosomatic: the mind affecting the body.

Before we proceed further, let us first clarify the term *nerves* as opposed to real nerves. *Nerves* is a poor word for anxiety, a state of tension and fear that may be either acute and transient, or chronic. That meaning of *nerves* will never be used in this book. Real nerves are the electrical wiring of the body. They begin either in the brain or spinal cord and go to all parts of the body, controlling muscles and some organs and glands. They also allow us to have senses, relaying sensations such as touch, temperature, and pain to the brain. Real nerves are how the "psycho" affects the "soma."

Anxiety is a state of worry, fear, emotional tension—these and many similar words are used to define it. Its cause may be rooted in reality or fantasy. It may be chronic and ongoing, or occur in acute episodes when something triggers it, and it comes in all degrees of severity. Sometimes anxiety is perfectly normal. If someone is pointing a gun at your head, you should be anxious about whether he's going to pull the trigger or not. This is not the kind of anxiety we are talking about. We are discussing the anxiety that stems from the complexities of our everyday lives, the tensions of civilization, our unhappiness and frustrations with our jobs, spouses, children, financial affairs. Some of us know the root cause of our anxieties; others are in the dark, the anxiety exists but we do not know why. Whatever the cause, the anxieties seethe and bubble in our brains like a boiling pressure cooker, and, like the cooker, when the pressures build up to too great a level, they must be vented. The pressure cooker has an outlet, a safety valve that lets out some steam. Our brains also have outlets. We can vent tension and hostility by acting out our aggressiveness, by screaming, by throwing a tantrum, by striking out at objects or people. This, however, is usually socially unacceptable, and often counterproductive, so we throttle it. We choke off those forms of behavior, our brains then having to vent through their only other outlets, nerves, the real nerves.

The result, then, is that anxieties can cause the stimulation of different nerves, in different individuals, that go to various parts of the body, or even different nerves in the same individual at different times. Some of these nerves go to the heart, the result being palpitations, a rapid heart rate that has nothing to do with any problem with the heart. Nerves go to the intestine, and we experience the venting of anxiety as cramps and/or diarrhea from a spastic colon. The most common psychosomatic symptoms come from stimulation of the nerves that go to the muscles in the scalp and the back of the neck, the result being chronically contracted muscles that result in tension headaches and a tight painful neck. I mentioned this in an earlier chapter. To help you understand the pain of a chronically contracted muscle, I recommended holding out your hand at arm's length, at the level of the shoulder, for five minutes. Sometimes it is the muscles between the ribs that are contracted, the result of this being a sensation of heaviness in the chest and breathlessness, which can lead to the hyperventilation syndrome (see below) or to costochondritis (see Chapter 12).

Symptoms occurring from these kinds of disorders are among the most difficult to treat. Antispasmodics that can quickly get rid of cramps from a viral intestinal infection often do little or nothing for a spastic colon. Analgesics such as asprin or acetaminophen that can relieve a headache from a cold often seem to do nothing for a tension headache. The reason for this is not difficult to understand. Most of the time when we physicians are treating a disorder, the body is assisting us. Perhaps it is better to say that we are assisting the body to heal itself. At the very least, the body is neutral. With psychosomatic problems, however, the body is the culprit, the cause, and is directly fighting whatever we are trying to do.

One of the more common, and frightening, of the psychosomatic disorders is the hyperventilation syndrome. So many people suffer from it, and so few understand what it is all about. It affects young women predominantly, but not exclusively, and can result in a variety of symptoms. As stated above, it begins with anxiety creating a tension in the chest and a feeling of shortness of breath. There is no true problem with breathing; it is just a sensation. The result, however, is over-breathing. We can breathe so much that we actually get rid of too much carbon dioxide from our blood. This decrease in carbon dioxide makes us feel light-headed. It also has an effect on the calcium in our blood, which in turn causes a tingling sensation in the hands. The tight muscles, overbreathing, and frequent sighing irritate the joints in our chest and we get the pain of costochondritis. That is a lot of symptoms, sometimes quite severe, and all from excessive anxiety.

The treatment of the hyperventilation syndrome, and other psychosomatic disorders, would ideally consist of reducing anxiety, if possible. Reassurance and the judicious use of tranquilizers usually helps. There is more on the treatment of anxiety to follow.

Sleeplessness is another problem created by anxiety. Some people toss and turn for hours, unable to fall asleep because their minds will not let them. Others fall asleep, only to pop awake a couple of hours later from minds that cannot remain relaxed. You should know which kind of sleep problem you have. Some sleeping pills remain in the body for very brief periods, and will not keep you asleep for an entire night. You should also keep in mind that if you use sleeping pills daily, they are likely to become less effective.

I think this would be an appropriate place to discuss the overall treatment of anxiety. Remember, this is from the point of view of a physician who is not a psychiatrist or psychologist. Certainly, the ideal would be to change those parts of our lives that are giving us excess anxiety. That is seldom practical or possible. If the cause of our anxiety is unknown, or not real, treatment by a psychologist or psychiatrist to make us more aware of ourselves, or to expose fantasy for what it is, would be ideal. That, however, takes time, can be very expensive, and might not work. What we are left with, then, is the use of tranquilizers and sleeping pills.

I have given a great deal of thought to the use of these drugs over the years, how they should be used, if at all. They are certainly among the most sought-after types of medication, and there are undesirable side effects. Aside from being unable to "solve" our problems, they can cause mental drowsiness, depression, and, to a degree, can be addictive, but I have found that circumstance to be rare. They do, however, relieve at least some anxiety.

There seems to be something of a war against, or at least to limit, the use of tranquilizers and sleeping pills being waged by some segments of our society, including those governmental. Speaking personally, some years ago I was "invited" to a seminar at the local county medical society. There I was, all alone at a big table, surrounded by representatives of various state agencies who proceeded to warn me of the addictive potential of various tranquilizers and sleeping pills, and to inform me that it was state policy to limit the prescribing of those medications to a certain number of months. I failed then to see the rationale for their position, and still do.

The fact is simply that the underlying causes of anxiety that make people need, or believe they need, tranquilizers or sleeping pills are not themselves limited in duration. Where is the sense in three, or six, or twelve months of antianxiety drug therapy during ten or twenty or fifty years of anxiety? Are we to say: "We know your problems aren't going to go away, but we can only help you cope for a few months?" Indeed, I could better agree with the total elimination of tranquilizers and sleeping pills than with limiting the duration of their use.

I see one more inconsistency in the limiting of the time of use of these medications. While it is true they can cause depression, and may be addictive in some, there exists in our society a legal drug with side effects so much more devastating that it makes a tranquilizer look like a sugar pill. I am referring to alcohol. The deaths from its toxicity, and on the highways, its effects on work and the family, make problems caused by tranquilizers almost insignificant by comparison.

I try to discourage the use of tranquilizers and sleeping pills among my patients, and I say that to you. Try to do without them. Again, they are not going to solve your problems. Often I will advise retired persons who complain about being unable to sleep that they should read, watch television, or listen to music during the night, since they have no responsibilities they have to be fresh for in the morning. There are those, however, who have chronic anxieties and who do benefit from tranquilizers or sleeping pills, and I see no reason to limit the duration of time they take them.

Once again, if your doctor tells you that your symptoms are emotional, or due to "nerves," remember that he is not telling you the trouble is in your imagination. He knows the pain is real. But he also knows he will have a hard time doing much about it.

CHAPTER 23

MISCELLANEOUS COMMON PROBLEMS

This chapter is simply a collection of items that do not fit in the previous chapters. It covers a wide range of subjects.

Dizziness is a very common complaint among patients, but most do not pay much attention to what they are really experiencing, so their doctor often has to guess as to the cause.

One kind of dizziness is simply a feeling of light-headedness. That often happens to people who hyperventilate. Sometimes fever can cause it. Another kind of dizziness is called syncopal. This is more severe than light-headedness. It is a feeling that you are going to pass out, become unconscious. The third kind of dizziness is actually vertigo. It is a sensation that you are losing your balance, that you are going to fall. In severe cases, you may actually see the room turning around you.

There are different causes for all these types of dizziness. Most are not serious, some are. See your doctor if you experience these symptoms, but be able to tell him exactly what you feel. Does the position of your body, movement of your body, movement of your head, have any effect on your dizziness? When does it happen, and how long does it last? Pay attention!

A stroke seems to be an almost inevitable consequence of living to a ripe old age, although it can occur in the young as well. A stroke (medically called a cerebrovascular accident, or CVA) means that part of the brain has died, just as a heart attack means that part of the heart muscle has died. There are basically three ways a stroke can occur. Hardening and narrowing of the arteries can affect the brain the same way it affects the heart and legs. And just as there is a gradation of symptoms from angina to a heart attack, and from claudication to gangrene, so is there a similar progression of problems in the brain. If the blood supply becomes insufficient, scattered brain cells begin to die and we see symptoms of senility, forgetfulness. If the blood supply worsens, the patient can experience mild and transient symptoms of a stroke as described below. This type of problem has been called a transient ischemic attack (TIA), or a mini-stroke. When a substantial amount of brain tissue dies, we call it a stroke.

A stroke can also be caused by an embolus. If you will recall, in Chapter 13 I mentioned that a clot can form in the heart, embolize, and block an artery in the legs. A clot forming in the heart can just as easily embolize to the brain.

The third kind of stroke is a hemorrhage. A blood vessel breaks and floods the surrounding brain tissue with blood. This is often the worst kind of stroke.

The symptoms of a stroke depend upon what part, and how much, of the brain is affected. For example, the death of a portion of what is called the motor cortex will result in paralysis or weakness of muscles. If the speech area of the brain is involved, the patient will forget words or be completely unable to speak. A stroke involving the back of the brain can cause blindness.

Leg cramps at night is a common complaint. I am not certain what causes them. I get them when I sit and type for several hours. As stated in another chapter, they are not caused by problems with circulation, at least not those I have seen. One of the more simple and effective remedies is potassium, especially if you are taking a water pill without a potassium supplement. One of the best ways to get more potassium without seeing a doctor is to eat dried apricots an hour or so before you go to bed. It works in many cases. If potassium does not help, there are other medications that may. You will need to see your doctor for that.

* * *

Many women come to me complaining of postmenopausal problems, either flushing or vaginal dryness. The menopause, the cessation of menstrual periods, is due to a falling level of female hormone. Do not, however, think that there is one sudden drop in the amount of female hormone in your body. There is a gradual and continuing decline, and it is not uncommon at all for flushes to come long after your periods stop, or even to begin a second time years later. I remember one woman who was well into her nineties when she began experiencing menopausal flushes for the first time in her life!

My advice on these symptoms is simple. If you can tolerate the flushes, do so. If you cannot, take the smallest amount of female hormone that will alleviate your symptoms, unless there is a medical reason to avoid them. When it comes to vaginal dryness, hormonal vaginal creams are very effective. If you do not care about having sex, there is no reason to use them. If you do want to have sex, but it is uncomfortable, you are a fool not to use them, again unless there is a medical contraindication.

Skin diseases are the province of the dermatologist. I have mentioned hives in the chapter on medication, and sebaceous cysts and fungal infections of the skin in the chapter on infection. All I want to include here are the common skin lesions that come with aging that so many patients ask me about.

There are three common skin lesions we get as we grow older, and they are harmless. Those tiny red spots you see appearing on your skin are called cherry hemangiomas. The thickened, darker, crustlike areas that can be peeled off, only to come back, are called senile keratosis. The little tags that grow and hang are called just that, skin tags.

Many times I will get a call from a patient telling me that he was stung by a bee, what should he do. Once someone called and told me that he had a mosquito bite! For most of us, an occasional bee sting is nothing more than an unexpected, somewhat painful, temporary annoyance. But not so for those who are allergic to the stings. People who are allergic must take very strict precautions, under their allergist's direction. An allergic reaction to a sting occurs almost immediately, and it can be devastating. If all you have is a painful or itchy lump, do not bother your doctor. Just wait until it goes away.

Most problems with the eyes require the services of an ophthalmologist, an eye specialist. Everyone should see one regularly. Glaucoma can cause a significant deterioration of vision before you even realize it, yet can be checked for with a very simple test.

Sometimes I will get a panicky telephone call from a patient who tells me he has to come in immediately, that his eye is bleeding. That usually turns out to be a subconjunctival hemorrhage. If a portion of the white of your eye suddenly becomes red, but there is no pain, no discharge, and no effect on your vision, do not worry about it. It is the equivalent of a black-and-blue mark and will go away.

The final subject of this chapter is the ears. There are three parts to the ear, and they are affected by different conditions. The external ear is the outside flap and the canal that leads to the eardrum. There is no skin inside your ear canal. It is a membrane that *must be coated with wax* to remain healthy. *Do not put anything in your ear to "clean" it!* Most of the time you will simply be pushing the wax back into the ear until you form a wall that stops you from hearing, and often you will scratch the lining membrane and get an earache.

The middle ear contains the tiny bones that transfer the sound waves to the nerves that give us the sensation of hearing. This is the place where we get the typical ear infection. The internal ear is buried in the skull. It contains the bony labyrinth, the semicircular canals that are our sense of balance. It is a viral infection of this area that most commonly causes the vertigo I mentioned at the beginning of this chapter.

CHAPTER 24

A REVIEW

The quality of the medical care that you receive will largely be dependent upon your efforts. If you enter into the role of being a patient with a blank and empty mind, trusting to doctors or medicines or luck to see you through, you are acting only upon blind faith. That is not to say that patients with that attitude are likely to die from some gross act of malpractice, but rather that there is a fair possibility that they will be frustrated. They may feel ill or uncomfortable longer than they have to, they will likely waste a lot of their time, and they will probably spend more of their own or an insurance carrier's money than they have to. On the other hand, those who step into the world of medicine armed with some knowledge of what is in this book will stand a far better chance of having their experience as a patient be as minimally traumatic as possible. Blind faith is really only something that should be applied to religion.

I tried to arrange the Part One chapters in this book in their order of importance. Let us review the main themes and concepts in that order.

Few people enjoy going to see a doctor. There are those who may find it as something of a social event, but for most of us it is an unpleasant and trying experience that we would rather avoid. The problem is that if you do avoid it, unreasonably, you may wind up paying a very heavy penalty.

There is a medical concept of the body's "reserve capability." We are generally born with approximately three to four times more organ or tissue function than is necessary to maintain reasonable health and life. We can be healthy with less than one kidney. A normal heart has the capability to pump far more blood than we need in our daily living. We will fight infection normally, and stop bleeding normally, with only a quarter to a third of a normal white blood cell count or platelet count. It is a sad "what might have been" situation when people, because of their ignorance or fear, allow some disease process to use up this reserve capability, ultimately presenting themselves to a physician only when they are suffering in the final stages of an affliction. I am not saying that you necessarily have to see a doctor frequently, but you should see one regularly. Do not gamble with ten or twenty years of your life.

When you do see a physician, be certain that you are seeing the right kind. You may think you have a high enough degree of medical sophistication to decide on your own that you need one kind of specialist or another, but you probably do not. However much you think you know about medicine and diseases, believe me, unless you went to medical school, there is far, far more that you do not know. During my years of being a physician I have frequently seen patients who thought they knew a lot more than they did. I have never seen the opposite situation. There is no substitute for having a primary care physician who knows you. See him first. See if he at least agrees with your opinion.

Remember what you are entitled to when you see a physician. You are entitled to the best of his knowledge and experience, to a reasonable amount of his time, to an explanation of what his findings were and what is wrong with you, to have all your questions answered, and to be able to contact him by telephone when that is necessary.

As can be seen from the order of the chapters, after understanding why you should see a physician, and after learning about physicians, the most important thing you have to do as a patient is to be able to tell your doctor what is bothering you. The inability of people to do this is an extremely common phenomenon, even to the point of patients' misleading their doctors, sending their diagnostic considerations off in the wrong direction. Do not stack the cards against you. Do not worsen your odds if you have to become a patient. Reread Chapter 4 and pay close attention to your symptoms. You will be surprised what an enormous difference just a little mental effort on your part can make.

When you do go to see a physician, keep a few things in mind. First of all, you are expected to be frightened and nervous, so do not try to fight it, just accept it. Second, you are not going to see God, only another human being who certainly will not be perfect. Use what you have learned in this book to decide for yourself if you have received appropriate medical care, if the doctor seems to have a sufficient degree of interest in your problem, and in you. Do not leave his office without thoroughly understanding what is wrong with you, what should be done about it, and having all your questions answered. If you are not satisfied, find yourself another doctor.

As I have stated, medical tests are a very important part of modern medicine, and, to a similar degree, they are overdone. I doubt that it would be possible for most patients, no matter how well informed, to prevent themselves from being subject to unnecessary tests. The malpractice and economic pressures on physicians to order and do these tests are extreme. It is more likely that your physician will reply to your questioning with a statement that the test is very important. Your best course would be to not argue and do as he says.

Remember that your responsibility to yourself continues after you leave your doctor's office. It is important that you understand the reason for any treatment he suggests, and what kind of medication he prescribes, as outlined in Chapter 8.

I hope the second half of the book, the part dealing with diseases and conditions, will be of value to the reader in understanding the nature of his or her particular problem. Please remember, however, that these chapters are a very basic and very generalized description. The great majority of diseases that exist were not even mentioned. Even with those that were, there are innumerable exceptions to the generalizations.

Finally, I would like to say a few words about the future of medicine. The scientific and technical aspects of the profession are advancing quite rapidly. Indeed, I see us as being on the threshold of truly miraculous breakthroughs in the diagnosis, treatment, and prevention of all kinds of diseases. Let us hope that our political, economic, and social institutions will sustain a profession that will continue to attract those most capable among our young men and women.

INDEX

193